REMOVE THE GUESSWORK

The Highly Personalised Approach to **Health, Fitness** and **Nutrition** That Puts You First

LEANNE SPENCER

Table of Contents

Foreword

The future is here, and we're so glad to be a part of it. The age of personalised nutrition has arrived with the fast-paced discoveries around the field of genetics, which is now taking the world by storm.

It has never been easier to gain invaluable insight into what people's genes say about them and how genetic information can help you to unlock your human potential. *Remove the Guesswork* embraces the DNA test and what it can do for your fitness, making it easier to inform your decisions when approaching your training and eating. The age of personalisation is here.

By drawing from other trends, such as wearable technology, *Remove the Guesswork* concisely shows how by moving towards focusing on yourself as an individual, by way of your genes, you will find it easier than ever before to reach the health and fitness goals that you have been so close to achieving but haven't been able to get because of the frustration caused by one-size-fits-all training plans that simply don't work for everyone.

Personalised fitness and nutrition is the widely-accepted modern innovation in the industry and this book explains how people are being empowered by such training, through the application of their genetic information. It uses real case studies to teach people about what they can expect from DNA fitness tests, and how to make them actionable in their daily lives.

If you are interested in how the proactive move towards exercise and diet can help you, and how using genetic information can maximise your results, then this is the book you should be reading. It is comprehensive and gets to the point of the why, how and what, with detailed analysis and an insightful look at a field of study that is burgeoning and constantly evolving, soon to become paramount when it comes to fitness and nutrition. It even goes so far as to forecast new trends that appear to be emerging. It's not just a book but a bible on how to revolutionise your life and start living in a healthy and productive way from the get-go, using DNA to change the way we view the world.

Avi Lasarow
CEO, DNAFit

Introduction

Are you frustrated by the one-size-fits-all approach to diet and exercise? Do you find yourself feeling overwhelmed and confused by the volume of information now available to us on the internet and in other media? Are you frustrated because you're trying different diets and exercise styles and they're simply not working for you? Do you have money to spend on your health and fitness but no time to make mistakes and guess what the best programme is for you? What if I told you that there is a way to personalise what you're doing that will lead to greater and lasting success?

Our lifestyles now are becoming more and more time-crunched. We're busier than ever before, and the demands of work and home start to eat into the time we have available for looking after ourselves. Increasingly our fitness, health, wellbeing and mental health is being marginalised. The internet and the smartphone have changed how we live our lives, and as a result we're permanently switched on and available 24 hours a day, seven days a week. It's harder now to carve out time to switch off and focus on ourselves than it's ever been.

We live in an information age, and it's never been easier to access a vast array of diverse content online. A quick Google search using the term 'fitness' takes just under a second to return 1,430,000,000 results. That's a vast quantity of information, so how do you filter out what's relevant to you? There is a bewildering amount of data, recommendations, advice and instructions being distributed to us all the time via websites, marketing, government guidelines and social media.

Understanding what we should be doing to help ourselves at a high level is relatively simple; we all know we should be drinking more water, less alcohol, avoiding sugar and caffeine and taking regular exercise. We are frequently told to manage our weight and that being overweight is both socially unacceptable, and bad for our health. What isn't clear is how we can do that in a way that works for each of us as a unique individual. The one-size-fits-all approach to lifestyle, nutrition and exercise is outdated and ineffective. It wastes time and energy, and generally results in disappointment and lowered self-esteem as one diet or exercise programme after another fails. It's time to start thinking logically and *personalising* our health and fitness efforts. We're all different. What works for me won't necessarily work for you. This book will help you understand how you can remove the guesswork around your health, nutrition and exercise needs.

I wrote this book because I experienced health problems and it took me years to try and resolve them through trial and error. I spent 17 years of my career working as an Account Director for large corporate and financial services companies. In 2012 I suffered from professional burnout, and was forced to take some time to re-evaluate my life and the direction I was to take. Burnout is a crippling and dangerous condition if untreated. It's usually a result of a perfect storm of chronic stress, poor diet, an over-reliance on caffeine, nicotine, sugar or alcohol, overwork, relationship problems and exhaustion. I left my job, and after a period of rest, I retrained as a personal trainer and set up Bodyshot Performance Limited, based in South London. Bodyshot was initially set up as a personal training company, but after listening to my clients' frustrations and seeing how difficult they often found it to hit their goals using conventional methods, and having experienced this myself, I realised that there must be a more intelligent way of working. In 2014 Bodyshot rebranded and created an ecosystem of products and services that offer a revolutionary new approach to health, fitness and nutrition. We work with our clients to help them exceed their goals by using their unique DNA and other health-related tests to create bespoke diet and exercise programmes. We work alongside technology such as apps and wearable devices to monitor and optimise the success of our programmes. DNA testing is a key part of every client engagement, hence our tagline 'Fitness is in Your Genes®'. It's an empowering statement, and a play on the uniqueness that underpins genetic science, and each and every one of us as human beings. Having successfully turned my health and life around, my purpose became clear to me; to promote good health and help clients prolong their healthspan by intelligently personalising their lifestyle, diet and exercise programmes. Whenever I talk about helping someone achieve longevity in life, I use the term healthspan rather than lifespan. The difference is crucial; your lifespan could be anything up to 100 years or more, but surely living a life that is healthy is more important than living a life that is simply long? Who wants to live to 100 years if they are severely disabled and mentally ill? Healthspan is what matters.

This book (and its title) is based on the framework behind my success: each chapter covers the important elements of health; fitness, mental health, personalisation, weight, our relationship with our bodies, exercise, nutrition, testing and self-monitoring, life hacks and lifestyle, injury and rehabilitation, overcoming adversity, motivation and inspiration and useful philosophies that will serve you well. The book is supported by personal anecdotes, client experiences and case studies that add a lot of richness. I have tried to avoid using complicated and unnecessarily scientific language, and I have included a glossary at the back to help interpret some of the terms.

Read this book and you'll understand what you can be doing to live a happy and fulfilled life. You'll be able to cut through the noise and get the right type of advice for you, and understand exactly how to make the adjustments you need to stay healthy. You will understand the principles of personalisation without the guesswork; what you need to do to give your body what it needs. This isn't your everyday guide to health and fitness, but a heavyweight book the contents of which have been put together from hundreds of conversations with clients and colleagues, to remove all the guesswork and get you the answers you need. Whilst some of the things I talk about in the book do come with a price tag, it is my hope that there is also a lot of content that you can apply to your existing lifestyle and training without spending money, such as my ten maxims for a happy and fulfilled life. I've really enjoyed writing this book, and I hope you enjoy reading it.

Chapter 1:
What is Personalisation

It's a very exciting time to be in the health and fitness industry, because it's undergoing a period of incredible change. There is now a huge area of opportunity for those companies and trainers who are forward-thinking and putting themselves in the shoes of their clients. I define personalisation as the skill or practice applied to tailoring something specifically to you. That means creating a fitness or lifestyle programme that's all about you, using data that we gather by a process of intelligent questioning, wearable technology and genetic testing. There's no guesswork, and no one-size-fits-all advice pushed on you. Personalising your health, fitness and nutrition reduces frustration, drives better results, improves compliance and works with your body to ensure you're doing the right things. It's as simple as possible for you to follow. Personalisation sits at the intersection of technology and personal empowerment.

It's a really exciting time for you as consumers too, because you now have access to cutting-edge technology and science that can revolutionise how you go about your daily life. You can track, monitor and analyse almost all your personal data, to make better decisions and prolong your healthspan. In addition, the number of data points that can be monitored and cross-correlated grow every year as the technology gets more sophisticated and more accurate.

It all feels very new, but in fact this kind of technology has been around for a while. Genetic testing for diet and fitness has been around for several years, and wearable tech has been around since at least 2008. What we've seen in the last few years though has been a surge in technological advancement. It's now possible to track sleep patterns, heart rate variability, calories, steps, activity levels, blood pressure, insulin levels, cortisol levels, and many other data points using small, wearable devices. In the past you would be wired up to machines in a lab to capture this data.

Personalisation is also known by other terms. The quantified self is one such term, which is believed to have been coined by the editors of *Wired* Magazine, Gary Wolf and Kevin Kelly, in 2007. Other terms include lifelogging, auto-analytics, body-hacking, 'biohacking', personal informatics and the rather creepy self-surveillance. I'll use the term personalisation through the book to avoid confusion.

It is my belief that personalisation will bring people out of traditional gyms and into the care of specialists, and the dieting world will either have to embrace DNA testing or risk being left behind. Anyone who is practicing in the nutrition and fitness space - personal trainers, nutritional therapists, wellbeing coaches and so on – will either be embracing the concepts of personalisation or will be looking for other work. It's as simple as that. If you want to know what's here today, what's coming, and how it can affect you, then read on!

Chapter 2:
Fitness is in your Genes®

I love this tagline. It's the tagline I use for my business, and have even gone as far as to legally protect it as I think it's that powerful. It implies that we all have the ability to be fit, that genetically we are programmed for fitness; it's what we choose to do with it that counts. The play on words with genes and jeans is deliberate; often clients come to us with goals relating to old pairs of jeans that they'd love to be able to fit back into. It is also a direct reference to what we now know about fitness; that we can understand fundamental and game-changing information about our fitness profiles by taking a DNA test.

Our genes are made up of hundreds of thousands of SNPs, which vary from person to person (pronounced SNIPS, these are a common form of sequence variation on the human genome. It is SNPs that determine our genetic differences). Each of the SNPs contain a genetic variation which reveals how each of us as individuals responds to exercise and nutrition. In just the last few years, technology has enabled us to tap into that data for our benefit. What's more, you don't have to be a top athlete to access this information; it's freely available to anyone who has the budget and desire to take the test. Understanding this information enables you to remove the guesswork around what you're doing, and understand what your genetic blueprint is for good health.

DNA and genetics

Human beings are 99.5% the same and 0.5% different. It's that 0.5% difference that's really important; that's the 30 million letters in our genetic code that make each one of us unique. Within the 30 million

letters, there are Single Nucleotide Polymorphisms (SNPs) that
I mentioned earlier.

We've known for a while now that our DNA is determined at birth
based on the genes of our mother and father, but that's not the full
picture. Our DNA can also be influenced by interaction between our
genes and the environment. Things like exercise and activity; toxins
such as pollution, circadian rhythms such as sleep, alcohol and drugs,
food and nutrients, bacteria and viruses, sunlight and vitamin D3 all
affect our genes. In addition, what forms our genetic make-up doesn't
just start from the moment we're conceived; it starts well before that,
with the diet that our mothers ate.

Recently, an experiment was done with animals to explore whether it
was possible to make genes in an embryo more active (or even turn
them off) by varying the mother's diet. (It turns out it was possible,
but ethics prevent us from conducting a similar experiment on
humans). However, a recent study in The Gambia discovered that
babies conceived in the wet season (whose mothers were therefore
subject to a different diet to that of the dry season) had different levels
of activity for a gene that affected the immune system (you might
have heard about this in a television programme by Michael Mosley
called *Countdown to Life*). So it seems likely that epigenetic changes
do occur in the womb, and what you eat and the lifestyle you lead
whilst pregnant can affect your child's DNA.

The Dutch Famine study

The Dutch Famine Study took place on a group of 2,414 subjects
between 1943 and 1947 in German-occupied Amsterdam. The study
was conducted to look at pre-natal exposure to famine on later health.
What they discovered was if you were a young embryo at the time of

the famine, (and therefore likely to be hungry and undernourished), you were twice as likely to develop heart disease later in life, and more prone to schizophrenia, obesity, diabetes, cancer and other stress-related illnesses. Alarmingly, there was also evidence to suggest that the genetic changes were passed onto the next generation as well in a continuing cycle of poor genetics.

Our understanding of genetics has progressed a long way since 1947, and it is now accepted that understanding our genetic make-up allows us to positively influence our DNA, to optimise our health and minimise risk of serious disease or even injury. It has also shaped contemporary thinking about how to use this knowledge to personalise what we do rather than following general advice which offers a one-size-fits-all approach. Appreciating that we're all different allows us to take more personal responsibility for our health, fitness and wellbeing.

The use of DNA and genetics in the field of sports science is relatively new, but game-changing. Major sporting bodies and clubs such as Barcelona FC (and at least four Premier League Clubs and three other European football teams) have performed DNA tests on all their players, and top athletes such as Craig Pickering (100m and bobsleigh), Andrew Steele (400m and relay), Jess Varnish (track cyclist), Jenny Meadows (800m), Dereck Chisora (heavyweight boxer), Glen Johnson (footballer), Greg Rutherford (long jumper) and Gary Roberts (ice hockey player) have all had their DNA tested to optimise their training and nutrition programmes. But it's not just for athletes; recreational athletes and everyday men and women will get as much benefit from understanding their genes as anyone else. As a company, we've performed well over 100 DNA tests with our clients, and the difference it makes is significant. Here's why.

Firstly, we don't need to make educated guesses about what works for our clients, and that makes things much easier. Our clients are usually very busy people; they have a reasonable disposable income, a really keen interest in health and fitness, but they don't have time to waste trying different diets and exercise programmes to see what works for them. The DNA test takes away the need for time-wasting and means we can write a detailed, comprehensive programme for our clients that is tailored exactly to their genetic make-up. No trial and error. From a fitness perspective, the test tells you what your power versus endurance ratio is; in other words, it'll tell you whether you are better configured towards power-based activities such as sprinting, hypertrophy training (high weight, low reps), squat jumps, medicine ball slams, and so on, or towards endurance-based exercises such as long distance running, jogging, swimming, cycling or lifting light weights. The test we use also tells you what your VO2 max trainability is (VO2 max is a measure of the maximum volume of oxygen a person can use – it indicates how quickly the body can get oxygen in and down to the muscles, and hence is a good indicator of potential performance levels). We are also able to determine your risk of injury (in relation to soft tissues such as tendons and ligaments) and your exercise recovery time (the time the body requires to recover from an exercise session). This information is invaluable for working out what type of exercise is best for someone, and how to structure their recovery times. Underpinning all that, of course, is nutrition.

This information complements the fitness data, but is highly valuable information in its own right. The DNA test reveals what degree of sensitivity you have towards carbohydrates and saturated fat, and whether you are gluten or lactose tolerant. It also indicates potential sensitivities towards alcohol, salt and caffeine, and whether you have a normal or increased requirement for vitamins A, C, E, D3, B6 and

B12 as well as cruciferous vegetables and anti-oxidants. Most of this information cannot be determined unless you've done a DNA test. Those who are particularly self-aware, and have experimented with their diets, might have an awareness of what works for them and what doesn't, but there is no real way of knowing without testing. Taking a DNA test will save time, effort and a good deal of emotional energy.

The science

Most DNA testing companies will examine a subset of your genes to generate a report looking at either markers relating to fitness, diet or your risk of disease. Some take into account individual genes, but most review a cross-section of genes. There are companies that will assess your whole genome, but this costs thousands of pounds rather than hundreds. Bodyshot partner with a company called DNAFit for all our genetic tests. DNAFit have a thorough and tested formula that they use to determine which genes they are going to examine. They review all the published literature available in the scientific community, and then rank that data according to relevance, sample size, reputation of the individuals who performed the study and of course, the evidence. They then establish the scientific validity of the gene against its interaction with the environment, and examine its links to the specific fitness or nutritional marker that it's alleged to relate to. Once this has been established, the company crosschecks that the effect is shown in multiple studies (proven, well-regarded scientific studies that have been peer-reviewed in at least three reputable journals) to ensure absolute integrity of results.

The genes

I am including a short overview of the genes that are looked at in the DNAFit test, but if you're not interested in the science or the specifics

of the genes, please skip to the next section. For those of you who
want to know more about the genes, please refer to Appendix A.

Angiotensin I-converting enzyme (ACE)

ACE is a small enzyme that plays an important role in blood pressure
regulation and electrolyte balance. Its activity leads to blood vessel
constriction and increased blood pressure. This is the most researched
gene in relation to sporting performance.

Adrenoceptor Beta 2 (Arg16Gly)

ADRB2 Beta (2)-adrenergic receptors are expressed throughout the
body and serve as receptors for the natural stimulant hormones called
catecholamines, or more specifically, epinephrine (adrenaline) and
norepinephrine. Beta-adrenergic receptors are found in fat cells, liver
and skeletal muscle where they are involved in fat mobilization, blood
glucose levels and in vasodilation.

Adrenoceptor Beta 2 (Gln27Glu)

ADRB2 Beta (2)-adrenergic receptors are expressed throughout the
body and also serve as receptors for epinephrine (adrenaline) and
norepinephrine. Beta-adrenergic receptors are found in fat cells, liver
and skeletal muscle where they are involved in fat mobilization, blood
glucose levels and in vasodilation.

Apolipoprotein A-II (APOA2)

Apolipoprotein A-II is a component of HDL and is associated with
obesity risk and type of food intake.

Fatty Acid Binding Protein 2 (FABP2)

This protein is found only in cells of the small intestine, the main site for fat absorption. FABP2 is involved in the uptake and transport of both saturated and unsaturated fatty acids.

Fat Mass and Obesity Associated (FTO)

FTO is a protein that is associated with fat mass and obesity in both adults and children, although its function has not been completely determined yet. Activity appears to be affected by eating and fasting. The enzyme is particularly active in areas of the brain that are associated with eating behaviour.

Peroxisome Proliferator-Activated Receptor Gamma (PPARG)

This long-named protein is a receptor found in the cell nucleus – PPARG is important in the formation and development of adipocytes (fat cells).

Adrenoceptor Beta 3 (ADRB3)

Beta (3)-adrenergic receptors are located mainly in adipose tissue and they play a key role in energy metabolism, being involved in the regulation of lipolysis (fat breakdown) and thermogenesis (process of heat generation using fat for energy).

Transcription Factor 7-Like 2 (TCF7L2)

TCF7L2 is a protein which binds to DNA and affects the expression of genes and the amount of various proteins produced).

Peroxisome Proliferator-Activated Receptor Alpha (PPARA)

Regulates genes responsible for skeletal and heart muscle fatty acid oxidation and is a main regulator of energy metabolism.

Vitamin D Receptor (VDR)

Associated with Vitamin D3 levels in the blood. Vitamin D3 is involved in maintaining appropriate calcium and phosphorous levels in the blood and providing immune support.

Alpha Actinin 3 (ACTN3)

Associated with a major structural component of the fast-twitch fibres of skeletal muscles. Only present in fast-twitch muscle fibres.

Peroxisome Proliferator-Activated Receptor Gamma Coactivator-1 (PPARGC1A)

Associated with the regulation of energy homeostasis, including production of mitochondria (an organelle found in large numbers in most cells, in which the biochemical processes of respiration and energy production occur). Also associated with fat and carbohydrate burning and conversion of muscle fibres to slow twitch type.

C-Reactive Protein (CRP)

Associated with a protein which rises in response to inflammation in the body.

Angiotensinogen (AGT)

Associated with vasoconstriction and blood pressure control.

Collagen 1 Alpha 1 (COL1A1)

Associated with vasodilation, blood pressure control, efficiency of muscular contraction and cell hydration.

Interleukin-6 - a pro- inflammatory cytokine (IL-6)

Stimulates the immune response to training and is involved in the inflammatory repair process.

Collagen 5 Alpha 1 (COL5A1)

Associated with Alpha-1 chain of type V collagen.

Growth Differentiation Factor 5 (GDF5)

Associated with a bone protein involved in joint formation, and with the Central Nervous System and the healing of skeletal, joint and soft tissues.

Thyrotrophin Releasing Hormone Receptor (TRHR)

Associated with regulation of the metabolic rate, mobilisation of fuels during exercise and also growth of lean body tissue.

Glutathione S-transferase M1 and T1 (GSTM1, GSTT1)

Associated with the removal of toxins, metabolic by-products, and free radicals created during the detoxification process.

Frequently Asked Questions about DNA testing

I've answered some of the questions I hear most regularly about genetic testing, and which you might be wondering about too. If there's anything that concerns you or you're curious about anything that isn't addressed here, send me an email at leanne@bodyshotperformance.com and I'll get back to you.

What happens to my DNA after it's been tested?

You post your sample to the lab for analysis. Once they have received the sample, it is analysed for about 50 dominant genes that relate to fitness and nutrition markers only. The results are then returned to the DNA lab and analysed. Once the analysis is complete, your DNA sample is destroyed. The DNA company scramble your name and personal details into an alpha-numeric code and hold your results in their secure database. Your name is no longer traceable, but even if someone were to get hold of your reports, the results themselves are of no real use to anyone with malicious intent.

Does the analysis reveal anything about my risk of serious disease?

No. From a business perspective, I am not in support of DNA testing for predisposition to chronic illness and disease. There is a place for it, and some people do request that information, but we don't get involved, and the test that we use does not look for genetic markers that indicate a risk of serious disease. There are companies that do offer such tests though, so make sure you check before you buy.

Will the test reveal details about my family heritage, i.e. paternity or maternity tests?

No. Again, there are tests that can establish paternity and maternity claims, but the tests that we use definitely do not. It is unlikely that you would accidently receive this information, but read the Terms and Conditions of your chosen provider carefully if this is a concern.

Do I have to repeat the test later in life?

No. The DNA test is a one-time only test and you can use the results for the rest of your life, making it a hugely valuable thing to do, with a vast return on investment. The only requirement for re-test would be when the science has progressed and many more SNPs are available for testing.

Do we know all we need to know about DNA for diet and fitness or is it a changing science?

It is definitely an evolving science, and that's a really good thing. We know quite a bit compared to a few years ago, but there is still a lot we don't know, and new genes are being discovered every day. It's a very exciting time to be working in the health and fitness world. When you combine DNA testing with wearable tech for example, you have a very powerful proposition. More on that further on in the book.

Have there been studies done to analyse the impact of DNA analysis for diet and fitness?

Yes. A very recent study led by Dr. Keith Grimaldi called the Athens Weight Management Study looked at a group of patients with a history of weight loss failure. The 93 participants were all taken from the same clinic and had similar characteristics (age, sex, frequency of clinic visits and BMI at the start of the study). 50 of the group were given a DNA test, and the other 43 were not. The study leaders measured their BMI at the start of the study, and again after 100 days and then finally after 300 days. At the end of the study, of the 50 who had followed a diet structured according to their DNA, 73% had maintained weight loss compared to 32% in the non-DNA group. In terms of BMI reduction, the DNA group had achieved an average 1.93kg/m2 (5.6% loss) compared to the non-DNA group who gained 0.51kg/m2 (a 2.2% gain).

Is this ethical to use on children and young athletes?

In my opinion, the test should not be done on any child under the age of 16, and then only with the consent of a parent or guardian. There is no legal age for DNA testing for diet and fitness in the UK, but the company we work with will not provide DNA tests to anyone under the age of 18.

Is the test intrusive or invasive in any way?

No. The test is an oral swab test which you can do yourself using the small swab stick provided in the testing kit. The whole process takes just a few minutes. The test uses saliva not blood so it's very simple to do at home. There are some conditions about when to take the test in order to get the best results, but the instructions are brief and easy to follow.

How accurate are the results?

This will depend on which test you've taken. The company we currently work with state clearly on their website that they have strict quality controls in place, and have a 100% accuracy rating. When I did my test, the results made perfect sense to me, and having subsequently made a number of significant changes to my diet based on the symptoms I was suffering from, the DNA results have proved to be spot on for me. I've also done the test with many clients with whom I'd been working for a while, and the results also rang true with what I knew of them. I personally believe the results to be highly reliable and accurate.

Can I still do the test if I am ill or pregnant?

Yes. Most tests use cells from your cheek, and these aren't compromised by illness or pregnancy, so the results will be accurate. The only exception is if you've had a bone marrow transplant, in which case you might have some of your donor's cells in your saliva, which could potentially contaminate the results.

Personalisation: getting the holistic view

The DNA test is a solid starting point and provides both you and us with your genetic blueprint for optimal health. However, what it doesn't tell us is where you're at now with regard to your health. This can be done using a number of other tests which we have found useful to personalise a client's nutrition and exercise programme.

Before we do any testing, it's important to us to understand exactly what's going on with our client, and the best way to achieve that is to listen, and then ask questions afterwards. Our typical client will present with any number of the following issues: stress, tiredness or fatigue, suppressed immune system, unexplained aches and pains, frustration at a lack of results, and weight management issues (underweight as well as overweight). What's important is that we find out how they're really feeling and what they want to feel like. Bridging the gap between those two realities is determined by the tests we'll do and then the subsequent advice. In addition to the DNA test, the other tests that we find are helpful include vitamin D3, adrenal stress, thyroid performance, basal body temperature, food intolerances and gastro-intestinal performance (GI effects). Here's a little bit more detail on each of those and why they're useful.

Vitamin D3

Many of us lack adequate amounts of vitamin D3 in our system. The only way is to find out via a simple, non-invasive test which can be done by a pinprick. It's a small plastic device that contains a pin and when you place it over your finger and push down, draws a tiny amount of blood which can then be squeezed onto a piece of card to be assessed. Vitamin D3 is actually a hormone, not a vitamin, and can only be synthesised by the sun, hence its nickname "the sunshine vitamin". There are such minute traces of it in food, there is no other way to ensure you're getting adequate amounts than by controlled and limited exposure to the sun. Symptoms of low levels of vitamin D3 include fatigue, muscle and joint pain and depression, and it's often an issue for our clients who typically work indoors in office buildings.

Adrenal stress index

The adrenal glands are located just above each kidney and they control the main adrenal hormone, cortisol, as well as the sex hormones. Cortisol, when functioning correctly, rises and falls in a pattern, and is a very good indicator of how well your body is dealing with stress. It's also important for the metabolism and utilisation of fats, proteins and carbohydrates. Cortisol helps to control inflammation and blood sugar levels, as well as having a large influence on blood pressure, nerve and brain activity, heart health and immune function.

The test is also a simple saliva test. At four set intervals across a single 24-hour period, you spit into a test tube, then freeze it before posting it back to the lab. I've had the test done and I'll share my results with you in the case study at the end of this book. This is not only a good indication of general health, but it also allows you to personalise your therapeutic nutrition plan to support the results. Again, it's simple, non-invasive but highly informative.

Thyroid performance

The thyroid gland is in the front of the neck and is made up of two lobes, one on either side of your windpipe. The thyroid secretes two main hormones into the bloodstream; thyroxine is the main one, and its primary purpose is to regulate your body's metabolism. The thyroid test is a little more complex than the others in that it requires a blood sample to be taken by a phlebotomy lab or at your local hospital by a qualified expert.

Basal body temperature

Basal body temperature (BBT) is the lowest body temperature recorded whilst you are at rest. It is best taken first thing in the morning before you get up or make any significant movements. It's taken using a thermometer which can be put in the mouth or under your armpit. BBT is a good indicator of how the thyroid is performing, and is a good, non-invasive first step before blood testing if a thyroid issue is suspected.

Food intolerance

There are a very useful set of tests that can make a huge difference to someone's health and comfort. If you think you have digestive issues, you can test to understand whether you have any food intolerances. This information helps you to personalise your diet and eliminate any food groups or individual foods that cause problems. (Testing for food allergies is a separate test – the difference is that a food allergy will affect the immune system whereas an intolerance won't). Many of us have an intolerance to gluten or lactose, and this can be picked up, as well as other potentially quirkier intolerances which might have gone under the radar for a long time.

Gastro-intestinal (GI) intolerance

This test is a stool test which you perform at home and send off to a lab for analysis. GI intolerance happens when the digestive system cannot process some foods, causing discomfort. Unlike a food allergy, it does not involve an immune system reaction – in fact, people with GI intolerance can usually tolerate small amounts of these foods without experiencing any uncomfortable symptoms.

I'll discuss how these tests can be used practically to help personalise your diet and lifestyle later in the book, but these are the main ones that we find that most people need. There are lots of tests that can be done, and you can spend a fortune trying one thing after another; once the tests have been done, the real value lies in the quality of practitioner that you work with.

Working with a practitioner

Don't be tempted to evaluate someone based on cost; like anything, you get what you pay for, and making a decision based on price is false economy. Go for someone who has the credentials and qualifications, and when you enter their name into Google, lots of credible and relevant content comes back. (In my introduction I referred to the vast amount of information that Google throws up, but be assured if someone is an expert in their field, Google will identify that and they will be easy to find). Ask for references and whether you can speak to one of their clients to hear first-hand about how they work. Once you've got your DNA test results, they're practically useless if you haven't got someone who is an expert in their field to interpret them into something meaningful for you. For example, my company only works with practitioners who are at the top of their game, and are experts in genetic nutrition. They have a successful practice or business, generate a lot of content on their area of expertise, and they are always looking to learn new things. Find someone like that and you'll be in good hands.

Belief and Compliance

One of the major upsides of personalisation is it helps you to 'buy into' what you're doing and why you're doing it. One of the challenges I faced when I started in the personal training business was around results, and how to persuade clients that the advice I was giving them would work if they stuck to it. I felt I was good at developing successful relationships with my clients because I found intelligent ways of working the relationship to get the right outcomes. If you have a coach or a personal trainer, the key measure of their success is how effectively they help you sustain your efforts and stay motivated during the time they're not with you, and that takes a lot of emotional IQ, as well as practical knowledge and skills. With or without a coach though, if you have personalised information about yourself and your body, I believe it makes it easier for you to stay focused and inspired to carry on because you know this is the right thing for you, not what's worked for someone else. It gives you belief.

Introducing testing

As soon as we started introducing testing into our programmes, things began to change. Suddenly, results started to come quicker, more efficiently and were significantly more sustainable. Our clients could no longer dismiss the advice as inappropriate for them. Previously, we were hearing things such as "I've tried every diet going but nothing works for me" or "everyone goes on about cutting out carbohydrates but I just feel tired and have no energy." The level of frustration we were sensing was palpable, and we shared that frustration because we've been there ourselves too. After we'd done the DNA test, we were able to put together a highly personalised plan for both diet and fitness, which was entirely predicated around your genotype (genetic make-up). Having this knowledge means you can really get behind the programme, because it's not shooting blind. The scientific evidence is there that states how you should be eating and moving, and this isn't just about weight management. What I love about the test is that it's all about optimal health, and for me this means weight management, yes, but also blood sugar management, getting the right balance of macro- and micronutrients, steering clear of foods that don't agree with you and getting the right quantities of foods that do. After all, managing stress and maintaining consistent energy levels is a huge challenge for all of us.

Locus of control

The importance of belief is vast, but personalisation is essential for creating that belief and allowing it to continue. Helping you tap into your internal locus of control is really important for belief and compliance. Locus of control relates to the extent to which you believe that you can control events that affect you. The concept was developed by Julian Rotter in 1954, and is now a key part of personality psychology. A person with an internal locus of control has a strong belief that they can control their life and what happens to them. A person who has an external locus of control believes that what happens to them in life is controlled by fate or environmental factors beyond their control. Having an internal locus of control is closely linked to a strong sense of personal responsibility, which is vital for being in control of your health, fitness and nutrition.

If you have an external locus of control, you may struggle to see how anything that you do could impact your health and fitness. You might find yourself blaming environmental factors, or bad genes for your lack of good health or fitness. If you are that type of person, you will probably see the most benefit from working with a fitness coach.

Stages of change

Prior to engaging with a client, we use a Stages of Change Model to help you to understand if our clients are in the right mindset. The Model was developed by Prochaska and DiClemente in the late 1970s, and is a process of identifiable stages through which people pass. The stages are: **pre-contemplation, contemplation, preparation, action** and **maintenance**. Often, by the time a client contacts us, they've already passed the first three stages and are at the action phase, but not always. Sometimes they are at the preparation stage but want that extra push to be fully prepared and ready for action. This is where testing can be very useful, as it helps us to ensure they are prepared, are armed with the important information they need and are psychologically prepared to take action. They will also have demonstrated their commitment by voting with their purse!

CASE STUDY: Anna

Anna has been a personal training client for over two years, before deciding to do the DNA test to see what other gains she could make by understanding her genetic makeup. Her story is a powerful illustration of how you can alter your mindset by knowing more about how you're built.

Background

In my mid 30s and single, I was going to the gym regularly and enjoying cycling and walking holidays. I was consciously controlling how much I ate and I'd almost shaken off the memory of being a somewhat unfit teenager with a tendency to carry extra weight. Then came romance and the pleasures of cooking and fine dining with my new partner.

Jump forward to 2013

I'm 41, have two young daughters and am struggling to find the time for exercise between my job and busy home-life. Inspired by a work colleague's achievement in running a half marathon, I join a beginners running course and make some new friends who help me to keep up my running even when the weather is less than inspiring. It is through one of these friends that I am introduced to Bodyshot, and I would say that it's down to both them and my husband's encouragement that regular exercise has become a core component of my life.

Looking for another level

To start with, my weekly PT sessions were focused on a goal of running a 10K race but then the focus shifted towards strengthening and conditioning my core. By the time I did the DNA test, I was training twice a week, and feeling pretty satisfied with the progress that I had already made, but I wanted to move it up a gear and find out if I was capable of achieving more physically-challenging goals.

Curious but sceptical

When I first heard about the tests, I was curious but sceptical. If I'm honest, I decided to do them because I felt there could be a psychological gain to be had - some hard data that I couldn't dismiss or ignore, and which could help me get rid of nagging self-doubt, and banish the little devil on my shoulder that would try to trip me up.

High sensitivity to carbohydrates

I did the DNA test, and I discovered I was highly sensitive to carbohydrates, and was therefore recommended to go on a low carbohydrate programme. (This in fact confirmed what I already knew from having successfully lost my baby-weight by following an Atkins-type diet). Having that confirmation would really firm my resolve to make the changes to my diet lasting and lifelong, not just a temporary solution to shifting a few kilos.

A big surprise

I had no idea what to expect with the fitness test, but my mental image of myself as being a slow but steady plodder - a tortoise with great posture! - led me to expect an endurance profile rather than power. The results were a total shock - I'm 2:1 power to endurance split, and have high VO2 Max training potential. This has entirely changed my mental self- image and helped me to feel much more similar, fitness-wise, to my brothers. Whilst neither of them ever spent time weight training in a gym, through their teens and into their 30's they excelled in power-sports such as rowing, rock climbing, and Olympic distance triathlon. I'd always felt the odd one out of the three of us when it came to physical fitness and certainly hadn't been as ambitious for myself as I was for them.

Personal empowerment

There was - and still is - something very empowering knowing I have the capacity to see a substantial increase in my fitness and that, if I put in the effort, I would see those increases quickly. Knowing I am not predisposed towards injury and that I have a good recovery profile is also very positive and encouraging.

My coach took me through both sets of test results and whilst it was up to me to decide what changes to make to my nutrition, they made changes to my training programme so that it now plays to my strengths and potential. Hill sprints are now longer and steeper; I've tried - and enjoyed! - track sprinting; HIIT and Tabata feature regularly; as does pre- exhaustion training. The test results have revealed a more competitive and determined streak in me than I was previously aware of: I really go for it when hill-sprinting with my training partner.

Other surprise benefits

One of the biggest changes to come about since doing the test is rediscovering my love of cycling. But this time I've had the confidence and curiosity to increase the challenge. I've competed in my first triathlon and completed a multi-day endurance event of running, on- and off-road cycling and kayaking in the Scottish Highlands. I've started using a smart power trainer with my bike and have already seen an increase in my power threshold after only a few months. Whilst I have it principally for training on my own, it's also brought increased variety to HIIT during my personal sessions.

Afterthoughts

Following the decision to give up my job, which I took at around the same time as the test, my health and fitness has been in sharp focus. It doesn't feel an indulgence: I feel I'm investing in my future and that of my family. I think much more carefully about our diet and nutrition, and am shifting the balance by having more vegetarian days in the week. My daughters see that it's not just their dad who really challenges himself physically: they see me training regularly, getting stronger and constantly pushing myself. Often they are inspired to join in! My goals for next year include a middle-distance triathlon and running a marathon. I know they will test me to my physical and psychological limits but having the knowledge about my genes will keep me focused on realising my genetic potential more than ever before in my life.

Chapter 3:
Exercise and Training

"The potential benefits of physical activity to health are huge. If a medication existed that had a similar effect, it would be regarded as a wonder drug or miracle cure."

Sir Liam Donaldson, former Chief Medical Officer

Starting an exercise programme can be a daunting thing, and most people give up in the first few weeks. It's worth spending some time talking about the common mistakes that people make, and giving you tips on how you can avoid them to ensure you progress towards your goals, stay injury-free and keep motivated.

Thinking you can do it alone

Being unsure of what to do is one of the biggest mistakes we see. If you're uncertain about what you're doing, it's likely that it will lead to injury as a result of poor technique.

> **TIP:** Hire a fitness coach or find a motivated exercise partner with some experience of training to help you.

Under-appreciating how hard it can be at the start

Starting an exercise programme can be very rewarding, but invariably the first few sessions are tough, no matter how fit you used to be.

TIP: Mentally prepare yourself. A great way to do this is to make a list of all the reasons you're starting exercise, and pin them up on the wall somewhere as a constant reminder. Perhaps include a photo of a fitter or slimmer you if that's your goal.

Ignoring nutrition

Exercise is just one part of the equation when it comes to health and fitness. Optimising your nutrition will pay huge dividends when it comes to weight management, injury prevention and general good health.

TIP: Keep a food diary. You will be surprised by some aspects of it, and it's a good first step towards introducing changes.

Overdoing it

It's laudable when someone makes the decision to start exercising, but pacing and gradual progression is vital to success. All too often I hear about people who've gone too hard too soon and are either injured or completely put off.

TIP: Start slowly and build up from there. Work with a coach who can plan your training for you, or if you're going it alone, try and end each session thinking you could have done more and work upwards from there.

Neglecting to stretch

Stretching is crucial after every workout. Most of us have desk jobs, which encourages poor posture, so our muscles are short and tight. Exercise can have the same effect, so stretching afterwards is very important.

> **TIP**: Schedule in 5-10 minutes of each day to gently stretch, as well as post-workout. Consider doing some yoga at least once a week for longer, deeper, supervised stretches.

Ignoring the bigger picture

I mentioned earlier that exercise was only one part of the equation. Sleep, a balanced lifestyle, low stress, good hydration, meditation and time to yourself are all equally important for good health.

> **TIP**: Take some time to think about how those things balance up in your life, and identify where you could make changes. Start small.

Obsessing with the Garmin and other gadgets

Personalised fitness gadgets like Fitbit, Garmin and the Nike bands are great if they encourage you to take an interest in your fitness, but sometimes they can distract from the pure pleasure of exercising.

However, listening to music can be very beneficial. Research conducted by Dr. Costas Karageorghis of Brunel University discovered that exercising to music can increase endurance ability by up to 15%. This only applied to certain music genres though, and tracks must be between 12 and 140 beats per minute in order to maximise results. His latest findings on the relationship between music and exercise were put to the test at London's Run to the Beat event in September, where music is strategically played at certain points of the course to enhance the runner's performance.

> **TIP:** If you use gadgets and monitoring devices, try not to look at them when exercising unless you have a good reason to. Download the data and examine it afterwards but don't let it distract you from the session itself. If you're listening to music, set up your playlist before you head out.

The importance of exercise

If you're reading this book, you probably don't need to be completely educated in the reasons why it's important to exercise, but it's worth spending some time discussing the effects that exercise can have on the brain, as this perhaps receives less coverage than exercise for weight loss or cardiovascular health. Diseases that affect the brain, like Alzheimer's Disease can be helped by physical exercise and lifestyle interventions. It is possible to reduce your risk of getting Alzheimer's Disease, but also possible to slow down the deterioration if you've already been diagnosed. This can be done by eating well, exercising, minimising stress, staying mentally active, and avoiding excess alcohol and smoking (although it's important to add that age and genetics will also play a part in whether you are at risk or not). Alzheimer's Disease is now described by many experts as a global pandemic, with one in six people over the age of 60 diagnosed with the disease, and 225,000 people expected to be diagnosed this year (that's one every three minutes) according to the Alzheimer's Society website.

To conclude, exercise has a profound effect on the brain, and is without a doubt essential to having a long and enjoyable healthspan.

Think of the brain as a muscle

The best way to promote brain health is to combine physical and mental exercises. This can be done separately or in the same exercise. So for example, you could go for a run three times a week and also do a daily crossword to stay healthy. Alternatively, sports such as squash, tennis or badminton which involve fast, tactical thinking and spatial awareness and engage both the muscles of the body, are ideal. You need to keep your brain fit and nourished in the same way as you do your body, so it's good to think of it as another muscle to be kept toned, stretched, flexed and nourished.

Exercise improves brain circulation

Despite the fact that the brain only accounts for about 2% of our body weight, it requires around 20% of our daily calorie intake. It's a demanding engine. Exercise has the effect of feeding the brain by improving blood flow and transporting oxygen and glucose, and then removing waste products as the deoxygenated blood leaves the brain. The improved blood flow also helps improve memory and attention span and so is vital for good mental health.

Helps to encourage neurogenesis

The supply of extra oxygen to a part of the brain called the hippocampus (responsible for learning and memory) helps to create new brain cells. This process is called neurogenesis, and these new cells survive even after you stop exercising. The hippocampus is especially receptive to new neuron growth after endurance exercise, which is further evidence to support the argument that the best type of regular exercise for most people is both endurance-based exercise as well as strength work.

Improves mood

Exercise encourages the production of neurotransmitters such as endorphins, dopamine and glutamate as well as generating serotonin (nicknamed the 'feel-good' hormone). All of these neurotransmitters help to improve our mood and make us feel good, which in turn can reduce feelings of anxiety and stress, and have a positive effect on depression or reducing the risk of contracting depression. I discuss this in greater length in my book *Rise and Shine: Recover from burnout and get back to your best*, and if you've read it, you will fully appreciate the power of exercise for mental health.

Reduces risk of Alzheimer's Disease

Improved brain function can reduce the risk of serious and crippling conditions such as Alzheimer's and Parkinson's disease, strokes and cognitive decline. Scientists now think there may be a link between Alzheimer's disease and type 2 diabetes. The theory is that people who have type 2 diabetes produce extra insulin, and that can get into the brain, disrupting brain chemistry and leading to the formation of toxic proteins that can lead to the 'brain tangles' commonly seen in people with Alzheimer's Disease. Regular exercise can significantly reduce the risk of developing type 2 diabetes by as much as 60% (according to a study from Cardiff University published in the PLOS One journal, 10th December 2013). Really, it's a no-brainer.

Neuroplasticity

This relates to the brain's ability to learn and grow, restructure, rebuild and reorganise. Neuroplasticity can be affected by tasks which stretch the brain such as learning a new language, learning to write with your non-dominant hand or learning the alphabet backwards, for instance.

As early as our forties, our brains start to shrink, but there are things we can do to slow that decline and stay sharp. Around three hours a week of brisk walking can halt or sometimes reverse brain shrinkage (atrophy) and encourage neurogenesis.

Other reasons to exercise

- General enjoyment and meeting people

- Cardiovascular fitness

- Positive mental health

- Strong muscles, joints, tendons and ligaments

- Weight management

- Improved sleep patterns and circadian rhythms

- Respiratory benefits

- Optimal metabolic functioning

- Work / life balance

- Disease prevention / mitigation

- Prolonged healthspan

Personalising your training

The immediate and obvious way to approach personalising your workouts is by hiring a fitness coach. As the title suggests, they should be the one professional that gets to know you and your body really well, and is well-placed to get the best out of you. It is my belief that can only happen efficiently when further testing takes place, otherwise any advice they give you is simply guesswork, albeit educated.

There is no way I can know what type of exercise you respond to best unless I either test your DNA, or we spend months trying out different things until we stumble across the type of diet and exercise that suits you best and gets the results you desire. This is a really inefficient way of training, and expensive! Remove the guesswork. Take the tests.

Finding the right coach

If you don't currently work with a fitness coach, then I strongly recommend that you do as you will get so much more out of the time and energy you put into the sessions. That said, it's important to pick the right coach. Choosing can be tricky; there are a lot of them, and most of them are making the same claims and declarations about rapid weight loss, strength and fitness gains and about how friendly, smiley and motivational they are. So how do you cut through the noise and find someone that's the right fit for you? To help you make a sound decision, I'm sharing with you the seven mistakes I see people making time and time again.

Making a decision based on price

The old adage 'buy cheap buy twice' applies to fitness as well. Be very wary of choosing a fitness coach who seems cheap, as in order to make a decent living they will have to be working a lot of hours; you will not get the one-on-one attention you need, and that person will struggle to be there for you outside the sessions if you need support.

Not asking to see their qualifications

Be aware that fitness coaches can get the Diploma in Personal Training qualification after just six weeks of study. They are then free to present themselves to the public as an expert, and people will trust them with their health. Not all 'coaches' are qualified either, so ask to see their certificates. If they don't have a qualification, then they won't be able to get insurance, and that can be a problem if you get injured or need to make a claim. The quality and integrity of the Diploma will also vary according to the place of study, as with any school or learning establishment. I qualified from Premier International, one of the most highly-regarded schools in Europe, and I only hire coaches from there as I know what standard they have been trained to.

Going with the person who claims to do it all

Anyone claiming to be able to do it all is not a specialist; that's just someone who wants your business. Look for a coach or a company that works with people like you. For example, my company Bodyshot work with professional men and women typically aged between 30 and 40 and who have a keen interest in their own health and fitness. They have a good job with a reasonably high disposable income, but are time-poor and frustrated by the one-size-fits-all approach to diet and exercise. We use DNA testing to create bespoke diet and exercise programmes that achieve successful and lasting results, and use wearable technology to monitor and analyse performance.

Not asking for testimonials and case studies

Any good and reputable coach will not only have case studies and testimonials on their website, but they will also offer you the chance to speak to clients so you can hear their experience firsthand. Some will insist upon it, to make sure that you are their target client, as well as the other way round. It's easy to put up quotes on a website, but nothing beats a conversation with someone like you who has gone through the process with the coach, and is willing to honestly share their experiences with you.

Going with the coach who offered their time for free

It's vitally important that whoever you work with places a high value on their time. If they don't value their time, how can you do so? When a trainer sets a reasonable price for their services, they are making a statement to the client that they value what they do, and are committed to delivering a high quality of service. They will also restrict the number of clients they work with because they don't need to work long hours to make a decent living. It's quality over quantity.

Not asking what the selection criteria is to sign up

A good and reputable coach or company will have selection criteria. If they don't, then the implication is they're happy to work with anyone, which means they're probably just trying to scrape by as opposed to really making a difference for their client. An expert will want to be known for the success of their clients, and therefore will be discerning about who they work with. Look for someone who clearly states on their website who their target market is, or what type of person they are looking to work with. I know coaches who only work with males between the age of 20 and 30 who want to transform their body composition in 12 weeks. These coaches will be charging up to £20K for such packages. I also know coaches who charge less than that but they will have very specific criteria about who they work with.

Not screening for a strong and relevant Google presence

I no longer meet anyone for the first time without first running their name through Google. It's fascinating what you find. I googled one prospective client to find they had recently delivered a TEDx talk in South London. I watched the talk online and gained a fascinating insight into that person before I met them. I've also googled coaches who have wanted to join our team and saved myself at least an hour of my time once I saw the search results.

Signing up for packages of five or ten sessions

The days of selling packages based on a small number of sessions are long over. Making a major decision about your health and fitness is a long-term commitment and a conversation with a fitness coach should reflect that. It should be about the outcome not the hour.

Whether you're working with a fitness coach or not, using your DNA results will help you to personalise your exercise sessions. Here's how.

Using your DNA to tailor your training

Many DNA tests will tell you what your power versus endurance ratio is; this is related to the type of muscles fibres you have, although there are other genes that are looked at too (refer to the Glossary at the end for a detailed description). Fast-twitch muscle fibres are well-suited to explosive power and speed, whereas slow-twitch muscle fibres are more suited to endurance activities. This is only part of the equation though. My power v endurance ratio is 53.8% power compared to 46.2% endurance. This means that genetically, I am slightly better configured towards power-based activities such as sprinting, heavy lifting and fast, explosive exercises like medicine ball slams than

I am endurance-based activities. Overall though, I'm pretty well-balanced between the two. That makes sense to me, because I play tennis and box (power and endurance), do sprint sessions (power) but I've also run two marathons and often do long slow duration runs with clients or as part of my own training (endurance). If you heed the results of the DNA test and want to personalise your workouts, then structure your training according to the power versus endurance ratio. Of course, if you love long-distance running, but your DNA results say you're 80% geared towards power, do not let that deter you from your goal of being a long-distance runner. You can still use those results to positively influence your training. Let me explain; for instance, building in some sprint work and kettlebell training (typically considered power-based activities) into your endurance training will help with your overall endurance performance. Mo Farah is as lean as a man could be, and no-one disputes he is the king of the short and middle distance endurance race, but he will definitely be doing speed work and kettlebells as a key part of his workout. (If you're interested and have a subscription you can read his interview with Danny Scott for the *Sunday Times*, 29th December 2013 online, where he talks in detail about his training regime.)

Examples of power-based activities

- *Sprinting and interval training*
- *Heavy weight lifting*
- *Box jumps*
- *Plyometric Lunges*
- *Plyometric Squats*
- *Slam ball workouts*
- *Kettlebells*

Examples of endurance-based activities

- Boxing

- Weight lifting with 3 sets of 20-25 reps of most exercises

- Distance running (800m onwards)

- Swimming

- Road

- Cycling

- Racket

- Sports

- Football

- Circuits

How I'm using my DNA to personalise my half-Ironman training

When I start planning any training block, my ultimate goal is always this: to get to the start line fit and with every expectation of completing the race. I've taken part in enough events now to know that measuring the success of an event based on how quickly you can complete it can be counter-productive, and also lead to disappointment. It can also cause unnecessary injury risks, and cause you to peak too soon. Anyone can set an ambitious finishing time target, and run a fast first half (I just have to look at my split times in the 2015 London Marathon for proof of that), but the real skill in these endurance events is careful planning around training and pace management and being open-minded about making changes and tweaks as and when you need to.

Using my DNA

Before we became a key partner to DNAFit, I took the DNA test to see what results I got, and to evaluate the product before we took it on. I was really impressed, and could see immediately that this was going to revolutionise how we worked with our clients. The DNA test revealed my power versus endurance ratio, my soft tissue injury risk, my recovery times and my VO2 trainability, all based on analysis of my unique DNA. It also tells me what my ideal nutritional requirements are, with optimal health in mind. In short, I have a wealth of information available to me that I didn't before. In theory, I have all the information I need to plan my training, and ensure that I get to that start line in great shape, mentally and physically.

My fitness results

As I mentioned earlier, I know that my power versus endurance ratio is 53.8 power v 46.2 endurance, which means genetically I'm slightly better configured for power-based activities, (although really I should be a good all-rounder). This means I will include power-based training such as interval sprints, HIIT training and speed work into my bike and running training plan, even though the half-Ironman is an endurance event. My recovery speed is medium, so I know I need to build in rest and recovery times into my plan. If I do two sessions in one day (which I do on Mondays), then I'll take Tuesday off to recover before Wednesday's session. I might use Tuesday to do some light stretches or some foam-rolling, but that will be it. My injury risk is also medium (this refers to soft tissue such as tendons or ligaments), so I will ensure I have a solid stretching and flexibility routine to minimise this risk.

Scientific Study

In an article published in the Biology of Sport journal, researchers in Central Lancashire spent eight weeks studying 67 young athletes. The athletes were divided into two groups; one group was given the DNA test and the other was not. Both had been tested for two different exercises prior to the test; the first was a counter- movement jump test and the second was aerobic cycling. The group who had trained according to their DNA results achieved a 5% increase on the jump test and a 3.9% improvement on the cycling test.

The highlights of my diet results

I discuss in much greater detail what the DNA test revealed later in the book, but the highlights from a weight management and health perspective are around carbohydrate sensitivity, lactose tolerance and my requirements for key vitamins. I am highly sensitive to carbohydrate, which means two things: firstly, I am more likely to store excess carbohydrate as subcutaneous fat, and secondly, I metabolise carbohydrates very quickly. In order to manage my blood sugar levels and weight, I should eat a relatively low carbohydrate diet. Of course, I know that I need to offset this advice with the volume of exercise I'm doing, but this is very valuable information to have. I also discovered that I am lactose-intolerant, which explains some of the digestive issues I've had (which have been significantly alleviated by cutting out lactose). I also know that I have an increased requirement for vitamin D3, anti-oxidants, cruciferous vegetables and Omega 3s.

What else has the DNA test told me?

The test has also told me what my sensitivity is to salt, caffeine and alcohol, and what my body's natural detox ability is. I now know what my requirements are for crucial B vitamins (B6 and B12) and whether I have any sensitivity to gluten or am at risk of Coeliac disease. When you look at all this information as a whole, you can see that it is providing you with everything you need to tailor your diet and train according to your genetic make-up. Since I've been using this information, I haven't been injured, my blood sugar levels are very stable and my weight never varies. I can ignore the mass of one-size-fits-all information and advice that there is out there in both the general media and fitness press, because I now have everything I need to personalise what I do.

Other things I will consider

Nutrition and exercise are only two aspects of my training plan. I'll also be considering sleep (eight hours a night ideally), and making sure that my room is completely dark and my smartphone is in another room. Consistently good levels of hydration are vital throughout the training period – glugging back litres of water a few days before an event will make no difference if you're dehydrated. Staying relaxed and rested, especially in the couple of weeks leading up to the event is crucial, and I'll be factoring in a massage every two weeks with that in mind. I frequently do breathing exercises to help me relax, and I recommend this as a great way to de-stress and take a few minutes to clear out your mind of any chatter.

Top tips for ensuring you're fit at the start line

- Sometimes less is more – ensure you plan for rest and recovery

- It's OK to skip a session from time-to-time if you feel ill, tired or mentally you're not up for it

- Listen to your body

- Use DNA testing to personalise your training and nutrition plan

- Use wearable technology to monitor and analyse your activity levels versus your restorative sleep and recovery (look out for the section on the ŌURAring in the chapter on Wearable Tech)

- Don't be afraid to go off-piste – by this I mean, you don't have to 100% stick to the plan – remember the ultimate goal is to be fit at the start line!

- Try and enjoy the training – it really helps to make the event a success, and stress can be counterproductive to both your training and overall health

What else can my DNA tell me?

DNA can also tell you your injury risk and recovery time. It's possible to get all that from a simple oral swab test. So what does that all mean? Your injury risk really relates to the vulnerability of your soft tissues such as ligaments and tendons towards injury. If your injury risk is medium or high, you are well-advised to ensure you include a thorough stretch and flexibility routine into your workouts, as well as being very diligent about warming up and cooling down. Your recovery time result is based on what genes you possess that enable rapid muscle repair, and some of us will have the genes and some won't. For those that don't, you will take longer to recover from an exercise session, and should therefore be building appropriate rest periods in between sessions.

Case Study

I worked with a client who suffered from frequent injuries. She was dispirited and frustrated by the frequent lay-offs, and starting to give up on her training goals. She did the DNA test, along with some other tests for adrenal stress and vitamin D3, and soon we were able to see why this was. Her injury risk was very high, and her power v endurance ratio was 24% power and 76% endurance. Looking at her adrenal stress response, we could see that her cortisol levels were out of balance, so she was waking early and not getting restful sleep. Her vitamin D3 levels were also low, which we felt were contributing to fatigue, especially in the hard sessions. Her recovery time was slow, so we put together a therapeutic plan which included vitamin D3 supplementation, a diet to support adrenal recovery, and a training plan that included more power-based exercises, a stretching and flexibility routine and regular days off. The injuries disappeared.

How to hit your goals

There are lots of things that can scupper your good intentions, irrespective of how motivated you are at the outset. There are also a few strategies that you can use to help you reach your goals.

Set realistic goals

Think about what you want to achieve, and make that your aim. It might be to lose two stone, run a half-marathon, or give up alcohol or smoking. Then consider whether you have tried to give up before, and if so, what stopped you making it happen. Write those things down, and then consider a strategy for ensuring that doesn't happen again. You might find at this point your goals or resolutions change: for example, if you resolved to give up smoking but failed in the past because of stress, look at what causes you to feel stressed, and address those factors first. Stress can be very damaging for health, and therefore is arguably as important to address as smoking. If stress leads to smoking, and you still have those stressful factors influencing your life, then they are what you should base your resolutions on. Put a timeframe on that goal, but make it realistic. Don't rush. Long term success should take precedence over getting it done quickly. It usually helps to set smaller goals, all leading towards your ultimate aim. See the chapter on Mindset for more.

Make small, sustainable lifestyle changes

Introducing radical new changes to your diet or lifestyle will usually result in long-term failure. Such sweeping changes might work for a short while, but are very hard to maintain in the long run. This is the reason why diets usually fail, and there's a whole industry worth billions of pounds that depends on that sad fact. Instead try introducing small alterations or adaptations, then a few more, until whatever you're trying to bring into your life (or get out of) will become the norm. The changes will be slow enough for you to have adjusted, to become part of your life, just something that you now do (or don't do). This is particularly important with regard to diet and exercise.

Enlist the support of family – or be prepared to go it alone

Depending on what you're trying to achieve, it can be helpful or sometimes even necessary to enlist the support of your partner, friends or family. Let them know what you're doing and why, and if they can help, let them know how. You won't always get the support you need (this might surprise you but not everyone will be pleased to see you making positive changes for yourself), but either way you need to have taken your decision for your own reasons. Be strong, resolute and determined. Other people might get on board when they see that you're serious but it's you that has to make it happen.

Go it alone. You don't need an ally

It can seem easier to find a partner or friend to diet with or try to give up smoking together, but this is a risky strategy, as there's a strong chance that one of you will be that little bit less emotionally invested than the other. If that person fails, it's far more likely that you will too. Whilst it's good to have an ally, it does lessen your chances of success, but if you do want to tie your goals to someone else, choose carefully!

Motivate yourself with something you care about

I helped a client train for and complete the London Marathon in 2013. She had never run before, did no exercise (in fact had never exercised in any significant way in her lifetime) and was in far from ideal physical condition when we started. Four months later, she crossed the finish line and proudly limped home with a medal. The primary reason that she was able to do this was this: she had a *very strong motivating factor*, which drove her forwards every day until she had finished the marathon. This factor was her father, who was and still is profoundly ill with MS.

She trained through snow, sun, hail, wind, rain and often in the dark three times a week for over 16 weeks and never missed a session. She was also very open-minded about making the necessary alterations to her diet to help her maintain her energy levels, and making significant sacrifices to her social life. In addition, she had a full-time job in the media and two young children at home. If you want to make changes then it really helps to have something to aim for, and something to fall against when it gets tough, because no matter who you are, it will sometimes be tough. This might be health-related or not, but find something that matters to you and start believing in it.

Why you might not be getting results

There are many reasons why you might not be getting the results you want and are working hard for. The best bit of advice I can give you is this: **listen to your body**. It's perfectly possible – and very common – to be doing all the right things according to your DNA profile, and yet still not getting results. So why would this be?

Stress

Here's the scary headline: stress is one of the single biggest causes of preventable death in the UK. Even when it's not fatal, it can blight lives and cause a lot of misery. Stress has an incredible impact on the body as well as the mind. Let's looks at the body first. Exercise will raise cortisol levels, and that's healthy and normal. However, if there are already elevated levels of cortisol in the blood, and you go out and do a workout, it can have a damaging or counterproductive effect. You might actually be damaging your muscles when they are not well-equipped to repair themselves, lowering your immune response and encouraging inflammation. If you're feeling very stressed out, you might be better served going for a light jog, a walk or just going home to rest. There is now a powerful tool in the form of the ŌURAring that amplifies the signals sent out by your body; more on that later.

Age

There's not much we can do about this one, except roll with the punches and accept that as we get older, we need to adapt our exercise programme and our expectations. The important thing is adaptation – it comes back to listening to your body, and responding to what it needs on a day-to-day and year-on-year basis as you get older. As you age, stretching becomes even more important, and be aware of prioritising quality over quantity. In other words, put the quality of the exercise sessions over the number of sessions you do and how long they are. That's good advice irrespective of age, but particularly important from around 35-40 onwards.

Goals

The old adage "what gets measured gets done" is valid here. Having a really clearly-defined goal will help you to stay focused, it's as simple as that. You'll still need to adapt and adjust according to how you're feeling on any given day, but keep an eye on your main goal and stay focused.

Sleep

Poor sleep can have a big impact on the success and enjoyment levels of your workouts. If you're not sleeping well, then your body isn't necessarily ready for the workout you're about to give it. You might get through the workout, but you'll miss out on the benefits if your body isn't able to cope, whether that's muscle-building (hypertrophy) or fat-burning. You can monitor your sleep using wearable technology (no need to sleep close to your mobile phone), and then cross-correlate your sleep data against your activity levels to understand how well you've recovered and therefore what kind of activity you should plan.

Hydration

It's very important to stay hydrated at all times. Note at all times, not just the few days (or even hours) before an event or a workout. Even when you're 2% dehydrated, your performance will be affected. Losing more than 5% of body weight can impair your performance impairment up to 30% (Armstrong et al. 1985; Craig and Cummings 1966; Maughan 1991; Sawka and Pandolf 1990). One of the biggest mistakes I see is people neglecting to drink enough water. I've heard all the excuses, from not wanting to go to the loo every hour to not liking the taste. It's vital to survival and optimum health: just find a way to drink it!

Your training partner

Sometimes your success can be affected by the person you're working out with. Are you finding that you end up following their workout, the one they enjoy and get results from? Is that person really supportive of your goals? It might be that you're better served working out alone, or just doing aspects of your workouts together. Beware of training with your partner, too, as that rarely works in my experience! (Although if it does work, great, stick with it.)

Case Study

I had been working with Jess for over two years, and we'd had some incredible results. She had lost two stone, had significantly improved muscle tone, her general health was much better than before and she rarely fell ill. Then things changed – or rather they didn't. We weren't getting as much out of the workouts as before, performance levels had plateaued and Jess had very low energy levels. She wasn't motivated or inspired by the sessions and she felt she was tired all the time and apathetic. When she turned up for her next session, rather than train, we went for a walk instead and had a coaching session to discuss what was going on for her. It turned out that she was under a lot of pressure at work, and also had a lot of coursework to complete for a qualification she was studying for. Everything had reached a point of critical mass, and the pressure of maintaining her exercise programme was too much. Rather than cancel, Jess was turning up but just making herself feel more stressed out. I recommended she take the next week off training to focus on finishing her coursework to a good standard, and put together a therapeutic recovery plan to help her get her stress levels down and support her body in what was a challenging time.

Chapter 4:
Injury, Recovery and Rehabilitation

Personalisation to avoid injury

Injuries are inevitable for most except the very fortunate, and can really sabotage your fitness efforts. I've had three injuries that have affected my training, and each time I've learned something new about how to cope with them. In fact, my whole ethos about intelligent training stems from my injuries and training setbacks, not from when things were going well. My first injury was a calf tear several years ago at the Men's Health event called Survival of the Fittest, held at Battersea Power Station in London. It's a 10K run peppered with obstacles, and to make things even more challenging, there are literally hordes of people around you battling to overtake. I was preparing to run up a 45-degree ramp when someone muscled past me, so I shot off even quicker and tore my calf. I wasn't a fitness professional then, but a City executive, and had no idea about proper warm-up. I also used to wear high heels to work every day, which will come as a shock to those who know me, so my calves were very shortened and tight. Not ideal for running up a platform of any angle, let alone at speed. To make things worse, the St John's Ambulance person was of little help, and didn't even tell me to ice the calf, so there's still a lot of scar tissue there even today.

The second injury was my left calf, but more recently, when I was qualified in fitness and knew a lot more about how to take care of myself. I was half-way through a marathon training schedule which included hill sprints, which I suspect had already started to put a lot of strain on my calves. Halfway during the training block,

I did a photo shoot in my local park, which involved lots of very short sprints but repeated many times in order to get the right shot. It was a cold day, I wasn't very warmed up, and I managed to pull the calf. Not wanting to take too much time out of my marathon training schedule, I rushed back and the pull turned into a tear. Not very clever I know.

The third injury was a result of an over-ambitious yoga move, which landed me firmly on my sitting bone (or ischial tuberosity to give it its formal name). That injury lurked in the background, not really giving me that much of an issue until I started doing a lot more sprint work, and then it really flared up. It has taken months of yoga, occasional osteopathy and foam rolling to heal significantly, and I still have problems with that and the hamstring.

For those who are unfamiliar with it, the foam roller is a great bit of kit. It's a cylinder-shaped foam object which is either smooth or grooved, and is used to roll out muscle fibres using your bodyweight. You can use it on all the major muscle groups, and the edges of the roller can be used to get into the more awkward muscles such as gluteus medius and iliotibial band, and some of the smaller muscles in the lower leg. It's not dissimilar to having a message, and is very portable.

Tips for coping with injuries when training

If you've entered a race and get injured whilst training, it can be hugely frustrating, but there are strategies you can use to manage this time-out and maximise your likelihood of being fit enough to race. Your ultimate goal in any training block though should be simply this: being fit at the start line. If you're fit at the start line, you're in a race. If you're not, you might never finish.

Focus on what you can do and not what you can't

Usually, there's lots you can do despite being injured. For example, when I had my calf tear, I could still do lots of other exercises aside from running and jumping. With care and caution, I could still do yoga, boxing, core work and swimming. I even safely managed a week's snowboarding. Mentally, you're in a much better place if you focus on what you can do rather than what you can't.

Surround yourself with positive people

Some people can be very negative and have a tendency to catastrophise when things go wrong for them or people they know. Don't surround yourself with people like this; it's just drama. Find positive people to be around, or people who aren't connected with training or sport. They'll help you see perspective, and encourage you not to overthink the injury or obsess about it.

Prioritise your rehab exercises

All too often I see people neglecting to do their rehab exercises. No matter how small or tedious they might seem, get them done! There's a reason why you've been given these exercises, and if you knuckle down and diligently do what's been asked, you put yourself in a much better position to make a full recovery and get to that start line fit and ready. If you've self-diagnosed or consulted Dr. Google, stop! The internet is a rich source of information, but should not be used for self-diagnosis. Consult an expert and then follow their guidance.

Work on the things you can change or influence

If you're injured, use the time to review other aspects of your preparations such as your sleep routine, your nutrition plan, your hydration and mental wellbeing. These are super-important aspects of race preparation which need to be considered well in advance, so what better time to review what you're doing. Also use this time to plan the logistical aspects of your race; your kit, travel arrangements, spectator arrangements, and so on.

Change the scenery

I find it can be really helpful to have a change of scenery when injured. Usually the weekend includes a long run or long cycle, depending on what you're training for. Take advantage of the training hiatus and get away for the weekend if you can. A change of scene can really help clear the head and take your mind off the race and what you should have been doing.

Don't rush back and flex the plan

It's the most common mistake I see, and I've made it myself. Rushing back after an injury or getting overexcited and overdoing it usually results in one thing: re-injury. Take it easy and flex the plan – by this I mean go back through it as though you were starting from scratch, rather than picking up where you left off. Keep doing the rehab exercises, and focus on sleep, nutrition, hydration and a good stretching and flexibility routine to support your recovery. Don't be afraid to ask for help if you're not sure what you're doing.

Tips to help you recover from injury

There are many things that you can do to minimise the risk of, and recover from, injury. A personalised diet and exercise plan will ensure that you're mitigating your risk as much as possible, and here are the other important things to consider.

Use your DNA

The DNA reports will provide you with your injury risk, based on whether or not you have certain variations of genes that code for structural and inflammatory proteins (collagen and interleukin-6). People who have experienced muscular or soft tissue injuries have significantly higher frequency of these variations, and therefore we know that these genes are associated with injury risk. This isn't a *fait-accompli*, however. We have known several clients who scored a high and even very high risk of injury, but have never suffered significant injuries. Cath Bishop, the Olympic rower who won Silver in the Athens Olympics with partner Kath Grainger, did the DNA test with us and her risk was high, yet she's never had any significant injuries in her career. If you do score highly though, you should be even more diligent about following the advice below.

Consider your past experiences

Have you been injured before? Can you, with hindsight, recognise why it happened? What have you learnt? I can see quite clearly (as I'm sure you can too!) why my injuries occurred. They aren't major injuries, but the first calf tear meant I abandoned the race less than two miles in; the second calf tear resulted in me deferring my marathon place until the following year, and the ischial tuberosity / hamstring injury has been a persistent annoyance (but not a showstopper) ever since.

If you've been injured before, it's likely that you'll have a weakness or vulnerability in that area, particularly if you didn't do any rehab or physio work. It would be advisable to do some prep work in that area before starting exercise or event-specific training, and of course when you do start, build up slowly.

Never neglect your nutrition

There are myriad reasons why a balanced and tailored nutrition plan should never be neglected, and using diet to support your exercise is vitally important. To help defend against the risk of injury, the body needs to be nurtured with high quality protein and healthy fats; an appropriate amount of non-starchy carbohydrates (and minimal refined carbs), plenty of water, between seven to nine hours of sleep per night, minimal stress levels, and an appropriate amount of exercise at the right intensity. I'll talk in much greater detail about the value of nutrition for all aspects of health, lifestyle and fitness further in the book.

Make time for relaxation and recovery

Make time for a long bath, a coffee with an old friend, laughter, something chilled like a trip to the cinema, or just spend time with friends and connecting with others. An unhappy mind is an unhappy body, and vice versa. If you're carrying a lot of stress, anger, resentment or fatigue with you, you automatically increase your risk of injury several-fold.

Make your training relevant to your goals

Injuries often occur for one of five reasons:

- Lack of proper warm up

- Wrong type or intensity of exercise

- Lack of fitness

- Overtraining

- Ignoring warning signals

- Re-injury from rushing back into training

I would never discourage anyone from trying new forms of exercise, and in fact cross-training is a great idea for keeping things fresh and working on overall fitness. Just make sure you're always properly warmed up for whatever you're doing, and do not be tempted to skip on the warm-up. I have a suspicion that a lot of people scrimp on the warm-up because they want to conserve energy, but that's a fallacy. You won't run out of energy by warming up (unless you are extremely out of shape!), but what you will do is ensure you're ready to exercise, the muscles are warm and all the connective tissues are mobilised and ready for action.

Ensure your training is appropriate to your goals

So for example, if you're a distance runner, there are some very specific types of training that will help improve your speed and endurance. Suddenly trying something new, that your mind and body are unprepared for, will increase your risk of injury. It doesn't mean you shouldn't try it, but be measured in your approach.

Intelligent training

Overtraining is a big culprit when it comes to injury. I've been guilty of it myself, and it's all too easy to do especially if you're training for an event with the deadline looming. I cannot stress enough the importance of *intelligent training*. It doesn't matter if you miss a few sessions due to injury, as long as you're fit at the start line. If you're injured, or have a niggle, and you push on, you risk becoming seriously injured and out of your race. Your only goal is to be fit at the start line. My second marathon was much harder work than it needed to be, because towards the end of my training block I started to feel the calf tightness again that was a precursor to the pull I'd had the previous year. I was on mile 14 or 15 of my last long run (20 miles) and I decided to abort (which I still believe was the right decision). I then had a long four-week taper, with very little running, before arriving at the start line feeling pretty good and up for it. By mile 16 I was really starting to suffer, mentally and physically. To make matters worse, I hadn't spotted any of the friends and family that I knew had come out to watch me, so I was feeling low, tired and pretty stressed. I finished of course, but the last quarter of the race was very arduous; much harder than it needed to be. I knew I'd cut the training short though, so I got the race I trained for. The trade-off was hard work in the last 8 miles in exchange for no calf problems at the start. The irony was the only part of me that didn't ache on the run were my calves.

Ignoring the warning signals is a precarious game. Quite often, it will be something that can be resolved by stopping and stretching, but if it isn't, you need to pay attention. If a niggle or ache is persistent, even after some gentle stretching and rest, then it might need looking at. Focus on your end goal. Very often, not listening to your body will just result in more damage.

Rushing back after injury is another very common mistake. I don't know anyone, at any level of fitness or athleticism, who hasn't been guilty of this. You have to be patient and allow the injury to heal, and not just superficially. It can take months for muscle strains and tears to heal, even tiny ones, even though it will feel fine to walk on. Give your body the rest it needs and it will heal; rush it, and risk re-injury.

Factor in massage and osteopathy

When I'm training for a specific event, I always schedule in a massage once a month (or more regularly if needed), and if something doesn't feel right I'll go to the osteopath to have it checked out. It's really good practice to go every few months anyway, as she or he might spot something that could cause a problem further on down the line. It's about prevention rather than cure. Again, simple advice: listen to your body. It's extraordinarily clever and will tell you when something's not right. All you have to do is listen. Think about that term intelligent training; identify where the weak points are in your body and target them, so that you can strengthen those areas before any vulnerabilities are exposed. Any decent fitness coach will help you identify those areas during a postural assessment and then put a plan in place to strengthen them.

Watch your hydration levels

Being dehydrated can weaken the body and that can lead to injury. Consume between one and a half to three litres of water every day, depending on your activity levels and the general temperature of where you are. A common mistake I see a lot is people glugging lots of water the morning of an event or shortly before an exercise session. If you aren't hydrated the morning of a session or event, you won't be no matter how much you drink. Hydration is a slow game, and you should aim for consistent levels of hydration throughout the day, every day. A small or medium-sized glass of water every hour is ideal. Another (related) mistake is over-drinking in events. This is called hyponatremia, or water poisoning. The medical advice issued by the organisers of the London Marathon each year puts more emphasis on not over-drinking than it does on the need to stay hydrated, because so many people overdo it. The right amount of fluids will help the body perform optimally.

Pay attention to the quality of your sleep

Getting sufficient amounts of sleep is really important to the optimal functioning of both mind and body. I mentioned before that I use the ŌURAring to monitor my sleep and it is not only incredibly accurate, it's also very revealing. I like to get between seven and eight hours' sleep a night, and I go to bed around 10pm or thereabouts. Despite that, I was only getting on average around six or seven hours a night because quite often I would wake several times during the night; the amount of sleep I thought I was getting didn't match up with the amount I was actually getting. There were a few things I could do to improve the duration and quality of my sleep; I put my smartphone away from me so I couldn't see the screen, and I limited the amount of hot drinks I had before bed so I didn't need to get up in the night. The most important thing for me though is making sure I've read my book for 15-20 minutes before turning off my light. Without fail that helps me to quieten the mind, and get a better night's sleep as a result. Making sure the body is rested, but more importantly the mind too, will leave you feeling happier, more relaxed and ready to go.

Personalising your recovery

Post-exercise recovery is as important as the training you do. If you've done a heavy session whether it's cardio or hypertrophy (muscle building), the workout doesn't stop there. You need to eat and hydrate to support the repair work that the body is now having to do. I don't want to get into the specifics of how much carbohydrate or protein you need to consume for optimal recovery as that's very personal to you, your build, what you've been doing and what your goals are, but there are some important things to consider.

Using your DNA

Your DNA can give you information about your recovery profile, and how to support the body post-exercise. My report tells me I have a 'medium' recovery ability, I have genetic variations in genes that are important for the removal of free radicals (GSTM1, SOD2), and so my report recommends that I consume a lot of anti-oxidants in my diet to support good recovery. The report also indicates I have a variation in a gene related to immune support and recovery (IL6), and to complement this I should include Omega-3s in my daily diet.

Your DNA can tell you a lot about how you can tailor your diet to support your genotype, and this is where the clever money is now. No-one I speak to is interested in the generalised, one-size-fits-all advice anymore.

Personalising your diet plan

Your food (regular meals), supplementation, smoothies and snacks can all be personalised for optimum recovery. If you can, base this on your DNA results to eliminate guesswork, but if you can't or haven't done the DNA test yet, then get some expert advice and then try things until you find out what works. More on what's included in the DNA nutrition reports in the next section of the book.

Yoga, stretching and flexibility

A great way to recover from an exercise session or training block is yoga. It's not only a perfect way to stretch out the muscles, ligaments and tendons, but it's also great for the mind. Yoga places a lot of emphasis on breathing and using the breath to move deeper into the poses, and this can be surprisingly beneficial in other aspects of life as well.

In the last 12 months, I've been doing more public speaking events, something I really enjoy. One event was a short talk to 20 sixth-form girls at a local school; I was part of a group of female entrepreneurs who run successful businesses in the local area. We talked to the girls about our stories, and gave them tips on how to find their path in life, and what worked (and what didn't) for us. That was a lot of fun. I was on stage again shortly after that talk, this time at a much larger event at a theatre in the Barbican. The talk was about the value of pitching, and the audience was made up of about 500 entrepreneurs from all over the UK. Despite this being the largest audience I've spoken to by far, I was very relaxed on stage and loved the whole experience. I had prepared well, but avoided over-rehearsing. I knew what the key themes were that I was going to discuss, but I had not memorised my notes so that what I said came across naturally.

Crucially, I'd been trying something new; breathing exercises. The exercises are really simple, but I found I had to practise a few times before I got it. You sit upright, and place your hand on your belly; breathe deeply, as though you're slowly sucking as much air as you can into the pit of your belly. Pause for a second and then slowly exhale, taking as long as you need to empty the lungs. Repeat, aiming for no more than six breaths per minute. I aim to do the exercises for 5-10 minutes each day, but settle for every other day depending on what else is going on.

I found that as soon as I started this pattern of breathing, I was able to settle myself quickly. It's now something I try and do every other day, irrespective of whether I have any speaking engagements coming up. I have done breathing exercises before making a talk or presentation, but I now know this is a bad strategy as the brain will just associate the breathing with the fact you're about to speak or perform, and it will trigger the release of adrenaline rather than have a calming effect. These exercises are not just for people who speak; they are useful for almost anyone, but I would definitely be considering them if you feel tired, stressed, anxious, frightened or under pressure. You might be surprised at how hard it is to breathe deeply to start with, but persevere. Once you realise the exercises work, it's very empowering to think that you've got that strategy in your armoury, and it can be used anywhere, at any time, alone or in company. Give it a go!

Chapter 5:
Food and Nutrition

Ask 20 people to eat the same diet for 10 weeks and you'll get 20 different results, despite everyone being under the same controlled conditions. This shouldn't really be surprising. If we put 20 people in an environment where they are all taught to play a musical instrument, we wouldn't expect all of them to be playing at the same level, even after the same amount of tuition. We're all different, biologically, physically and intellectually.

One size does not fit all

With that in mind, why do we still sign up to diets that follow the 'one-size-fits-all' approach? Wouldn't it make more sense to personalise what we do, in terms of both diet and exercise? Here are other factors that you should be thinking of when personalising your diet.

The over-simplification of 'eat less and move more'

What we understand about weight loss and calorie management has changed dramatically over the last few years, although this information is slow to filter down, in part due to media reporting and advertising. We are still recovering from the brainwashing we received in the 1970s about fat being the source of all our weight problems, leaving us thinking it's the macronutrient to be avoided at all costs. Actually, what scientists are now discovering about why some of us struggle with our weight, blows the 'eat less and move more' and fat demonisation theory out of the water. Here's why.

It's in your genes

Scientists now understand that how we respond to basic nutrition relies a good deal on our genetics. Dr. Claude Bouchard, faculty fellow at the Texas A&M University, says "the response to environmental, social and behavioural factors is conditioned on the genotype of an individual. Your adaptation to a diet or a given amount of exercise is determined by your genes."

It is believed that one day, medical treatments will be created bespoke for us according to our genetic make-up, and it has been possible for a few years now to buy a DNA test which tells you the best type of exercise for you and your ideal diet type. Other factors such as your gastro-intestinal health and the microflora in your gut also have a profound impact on how you process food, absorb micronutrients and store fat.

The obesegenicity of the environment

The term 'obesegenicity' is the term used to describe how the environment contributes to obesity. In the West, our environment is set up to be as efficient as possible; we have multi-transport systems which remove the need for walking; we have fewer outdoor spaces and fewer pavements; there are fast food outlets everywhere, usually rich in refined carbohydrates; many of our jobs are now desk-bound; we have labour-saving devices which minimise our need to move; our food shopping can be ordered online and delivered straight to our kitchens; our factories and machines emit toxic gases and pollutants which disrupt our hormone profile and in turn can affect our weight.

Social factors

It's become commonplace to prioritise price over provenance with foods, and we end up eating cheap foods that are not as nutritious. Many of us are now used to eating on the run or in front of the TV, and consume processed foods because they're quick to prepare. We're losing the love of home cooking and all because it just takes a bit of time. We need to value our health enough to spend that extra half-hour on a meal. Society has also normalised outsize portions - fast food and drinks sizes have risen year on year. The supermarkets are always running promotions on supersize bags of crisps, chocolates and biscuits, and people buy them because we can't resist a bargain (and product placement has something to do with it as well). It's even got to the point where people of a normal weight are being touted as thin because so many of us are now overweight, that's become the new normal.

Behavioural factors

Linked with social factors, there are a number of behavioural factors that affect weight management. We are now more sedentary, and less disposed to walk than we once were. We have become more reliant on transport and labour-saving devices. Many of us have a powerful cognitive dissonance, so even though we know we should move more, or perhaps leave the train a few stops earlier and walk the rest of the way, we don't. We often drink more alcohol than we should, or postpone the visit to the gym, even though we know we should be doing it. There is an increasing reliance on medications now too which can have an impact on weight. The contraceptive pill is commonly known to cause weight gain in some women, and many anti-depressants and anxiety drugs also cause weight fluctuations.

Our decision to take these medicines affects how we store fat and burn energy.

Calories in versus calories out

Traditionally, a calorie has been seen as a calorie no matter whether it comes from fat, protein or carbohydrate. We now know this not only to be oversimplified, but also inaccurate. The energy cost of digesting, absorbing and metabolising each of the macronutrients varies from each (although not by much), but the nutritional value of each can vary much more significantly. Not only is each macronutrient processed differently, but individually we will process foods differently depending on our genes and our gut flora. I've taken a DNA test to establish the best type of diet for me, so I know that I am highly sensitive to carbohydrates. This means I am likely to convert carbohydrates into a higher number of calories and I am also more likely to store excess carbohydrate as subcutaneous fat. There's lots to be said on this subject, but if you're unsure, take the test and remember, calorie-restricted diets won't work in the long-term. A calorie is not a calorie.

Intelligent training has moved on from one-size-fits-all

Successful weight management is highly individualised and what works for one person may not work at all for another. The simplest way to look at this is to think about what you know of yourself, and then consult a health expert who can help you mesh that self-knowledge with the results of tests and then some easy-to-follow advice. The sorts of tests I recommend include potential food intolerances, gastrointestinal health, DNA (for diet and exercise not risk of disease), vitamin D3, and adrenal stress. The health expert will ask you a series of questions about your lifestyle, medications, allergies and sleep routine to form a picture before delivering your results and recommendations.

Personalisation is the future

I've been saying it for a while; personalisation is the key to success in fitness and weight management. The weight loss industry is expected to be valued at £220 billion by 2017. Let's not contribute any more hard-earned pounds to these behemoth companies in an effort to shed physical pounds. Be smart about your weight management, and make it personal.

Using your DNA to personalise your nutrition plan

Using your DNA to understand the best type of diet for you is an ideal place to start. The science that supports this kind of testing is now very accurate, and an awareness of nutrigenomics is increasing all the time. There's been a lot of press coverage in fitness magazines and broadsheet newspapers, and many celebrities and athletes have done the tests and are using the knowledge to better their performance. Well-known nutritionist Ian Marber took the test and followed the advice for a year, and despite his initial scepticism, wrote a piece in The Telegraph about how impressed he was and what benefits he noticed ('What to Eat Now: Foods to suit your DNA', *Daily Telegraph*, 9th March 2015).

There are a range of nutritional markers that are covered depending on what test you do, but here are the results I got from my DNA test and how I've used them to improve my diet and nutrition.

Carbohydrate sensitivity

The DNA test will tell you what degree of sensitivity you have towards carbohydrates. This relates to three things: how quickly you convert carbs into calories, how likely you are to convert excess carbs into subcutaneous fat, and finally whether you tend to convert carbs into higher calories more than others might. I think it's one of the most important markers, because many of us are highly sensitive to carbs (in particular refined carbs) and should therefore be following a low carb diet. Having done a 30-day elimination diet where I cut out all carbohydrates except vegetables (and even then restricted to non-starchy carbs), I can personally vouch for the fact that much of our diet is now comprised of refined or starchy carbs. We've become very reliant on them for meals, and especially snacks. There isn't a café, bistro, coffee shop or fast food restaurant that offers much alternative to refined carbs, as I discovered. It's generally accepted now by thought leaders in the world of nutrition that it's carbs we should be watching (not demonising), rather than fat. (Read Gary Taubes' *Why We Get Fat* or *The Diet Delusion* if you want to know more.) People who struggle to manage their weight are usually consuming too many refined carbs, and will probably also be highly sensitive to them but probably don't know it because they haven't tested their DNA. It can be a game-changing element of a solid nutrition plan if adaptations are made.

> **Case Study**
>
> I started working with Diane in late 2015. She was several stone overweight, tired, unhappy, her joints were giving up on her and her diet was out of control. Her busy lifestyle meant food was often eaten on the move but she also frequently skipped main meals, snacking instead on junk food. We did the DNA test at the start of our working relationship, and her results showed that she was highly sensitive to carbohydrates. We focused on this as the key part of her diet that needed to be addressed. We worked out a diet plan that eliminated all refined carbs, replacing them instead with protein and healthy fats. Because of this high sensitivity, we knew that this was one of the root causes of her persistent weight gain, and explained the energy management issues she was experiencing. Once we had agreed on a diet plan that eliminated refined carbs and built in an exercise program consisting of at least two sessions of high intensity exercise combined with weekly Pilates. After six months, Diane had lost a remarkable 28kg of body weight.

Saturated fat sensitivity

This relates to how quickly you absorb saturated fat, which is typically found in chocolate, cakes, biscuits, butter and also animal fats that are solid at room temperature. Those that are very sensitive are advised to limit the amount of saturated fat to either the recommended daily allowance (RDA) or less. Fat has long been demonised as the macronutrient to be avoided at all costs, however, we need an element of saturated fat in our diets. Despite this, it's wise to be cautious about the source, provenance and of course, quantities.

Lactose Intolerance

Lactose is a sugar found in milk and some dairy products. Lactose intolerance is a common digestive complaint, but can be very uncomfortable and cause quite distressing effects for those who suffer from it. The body digests lactose using an enzyme called lactase, which breaks lactose into two sugars called glucose and galactose which can be easily absorbed into the bloodstream. The issue is that many people stop producing lactase as an adult, so the lactose stays in the digestive system where it is fermented by bacteria, causing gas and other symptoms. The DNA test identifies whether you hold the gene for lactase persistence, and so indicates whether you are tolerant or not. I've found that cutting out dairy from my diet resolved a number of digestive complaints, and has been very worthwhile. There's never been a better time to personalise your diet either, with so many decent alternatives to dairy on the market including unfermented soya milk (although not without controversy because it has often been genetically modified and contains phytoestrogens which can disrupt hormone function), almond milk and my favourite, coconut milk. Refer to my case study for more information on the negative impact of lactose for the intolerant.

Coeliac predisposition (or gluten sensitivity)

This often surprises people, and sometimes the symptoms of gluten intolerance are mistaken for lactose intolerance, and vice versa. Gluten sensitivity relates to the body's ability to digest wheat, barley and rye. For some people, it's a mild insensitivity, whereas for others it can be a real problem. If you have Coeliac Disease, the ramifications of consuming, or even being close to gluten, can be very dangerous. Coeliac Disease is an auto-immune condition, where the body's immune system attacks itself when gluten is consumed. This causes damage to the lining of the gut and means that the body cannot properly absorb nutrients from food. If you are not Coeliac but are highly sensitive to gluten, it is still advisable to cut gluten out of your diet. This requires planning and research however; gluten is an insidious ingredient in that you'll find it everywhere, even where you wouldn't expect to, such as in sauces, soup bases, thickeners, salad dressings, processed cereals and even ice cream.

Case Study

Jo is a deputy head teacher in her late thirties working in a busy school in London. During the consultation process, Jo described some difficult digestive issues that she'd been suffering from for a long time. She also felt frustrated that she was unable to shift a layer of belly fat from her middle despite exercising three times a week. Jo's theory was that she was lactose intolerant, and so she had completely eliminated lactose from her diet, but was unhappy about this as she missed foods like cheese and yoghurt. We did the DNA test, and to her surprise, she was lactose tolerant but highly sensitive to gluten. We eliminated gluten for 14 days and her symptoms of bloating and gas disappeared. We brought lactose back in, and the symptoms didn't reappear. For Jo, this was well-worth the investment because she finally got to the bottom of what was wrong, the belly fat also disappeared, and she felt back in control of her body.

Salt, caffeine and alcohol sensitivity

We all metabolise foods, liquids and chemicals in different ways and at different speeds. How we do this can impact important systems in the body such as our ability to absorb nutrients, or our ability to clear the system of unwanted toxins. Our DNA can tell us a lot about how sensitive we are and how we metabolise foods.

A sensitivity to salt is important because too much salt can lead to hypertension, (high blood pressure). Certain ethnic groups and individuals are more predisposed to hypertension, so it's important to understand how you metabolise salt and therefore how much of it you consume. The recommended daily allowance (RDA) is 6 grams per day, but this generalised advice might not work if you are highly sensitive to salt and have a family history of high blood pressure, for example. I have a raised sensitivity to salt, so I am careful not to add much to my food or plate, but more importantly I am careful about foods I eat which might have high amounts of added salt. This is particularly the case for processed and packaged foods. Salt has been used as a preservative since ancient times, so it's safe to say anything with a longer shelf life than it would have if it was fresh has got a lot of salt in it.

The sensitivity to caffeine relates to whether you're a fast or slow metaboliser of caffeine. I am a slow metaboliser, so I used to drink just one or maximum two cups of coffee a day, and both in the morning. In the summer of last year, I started to feel very unsettled after drinking coffee, so I've subsequently given up caffeine and now drink decaf coffee. It still feels like a treat to me, and an enjoyable part of my morning ritual. If you're a fast metaboliser, the caffeine doesn't stay in your bloodstream for as long, and you can potentially afford to drink caffeine later in the day or more of it if you choose. However, too much caffeine can cause jitters, palpitations, sweating and increased heartrate, all of which can be unpleasant, and it can also inhibit the absorption of certain vitamins and minerals. Drinking caffeine at the same time as ingesting calcium (perhaps in a morning multivitamin tablet) will significantly reduce the dose of calcium that is ingested (one source quoted that for every 150mg ingested, up to 5mg was lost in urine due to caffeine). Caffeine also inhibits the amount of calcium ingested by the intestinal tract, which depletes the amount absorbed in the bones. Linked to this, caffeine has the effect of inhibiting the vitamin D receptors which also affects bone density, and can increase the risk of osteoporosis (particularly in post-menopausal women). Drinking caffeine at the same time as consuming iron can reduce absorption by as much as 80%, so it's prudent to separate caffeine from a multivitamin or iron tablet by an hour to ensure the iron intake is unaffected. Because caffeine is a diuretic, some of the water soluble B vitamins are depleted in fluid loss, and excess caffeine can reduce the absorption of manganese, zinc and copper, and increase the excretion of magnesium, potassium, sodium and phosphate. All that said, one or maybe two cups a day is unlikely to cause any harm, but knowing your genetic sensitivities helps you to make an informed decision based on you and not the generalised advice.

Alcohol sensitivity relates especially to whether you are a slow or fast metaboliser of alcohol, and whether you possess a certain version of a gene called ADH1C. People who are slow metabolisers of alcohol will have this gene variation, and therefore a small amount of alcohol (such as a 175ml of wine or half a pint of beer or lager), will have a positive effect on good cholesterol (high density lipoprotein or HDL). Of course this doesn't mean you should start drinking every day if you don't currently, as there are many other ways to positively affect cholesterol, but this is the upside of being a slow metaboliser of alcohol and a light drinker. The downside, of course, is that you are more likely to suffer from hangovers!

Antioxidant requirements

Antioxidants are molecules that inhibit the oxidation of other molecules. Oxidation refers to the process of a chemical reaction. It can produce the spontaneous release of what are called free radicals, which can be cell-damaging. Antioxidants can stop these chain reactions from occurring, hence they are vitally important in our diet. The main sources are vitamins A, C and E, which broadly speaking can be found in brightly- coloured vegetables such as kale, spinach, chard, sweet potato, asparagus, bell peppers, broccoli, parsley, cauliflower and fruits such as strawberries, oranges, kiwis and cranberries. You can pack a lot of these foods into a morning smoothie. I use a Nutribullet to blend mine as it's incredibly easy to clean afterwards and the cyclonic action of the 600-watt motor pulverises the fruits and vegetables, leaving a smooth liquid with all the vitamins and minerals released and easy to drink. The DNA results will tell you whether you have a normal or a raised requirement for antioxidants, so you can refine your intake accordingly. The normal requirement for antioxidants (the Recommended Daily Allowance) is vitamin A (0.7mg for men and 0.6mg for women), vitamin C (40mg for both men and women), and vitamin E (4mg for men and 3mg for women). If you have a raised requirement, it's advisable to increase your intake by 10- 25%, and preferably within food itself, rather than via supplementation.

Omega-3 fatty acids

Omega 3 fatty acids are most commonly found in oily fish such as salmon, mackerel, sardines and so on. They are especially important for heart health and their anti-inflammatory properties, and even more so if you are pregnant. As well as oily fish, you can find Omega 3 fatty acids in flaxseeds and walnuts, and flaxseed oil. The recommended daily allowance for Omega 3 is one to two portions of oily fish a week, and if you have a raised genetic requirement, two to three portions per week is ideal, or alternatively if you are vegan or can't get access to quality fish, or just want more variety of options, you could substitute with flax or chia seeds in a smoothie or sprinkled on yoghurt or breakfast cereal.

Requirements for vitamins B6 and B12

Sources of B6 include turkey, salmon, beef, sweet potato, chicken and spinach, and the role of this vitamin is to allow the body to use and store energy from protein and carbohydrates in food, and to help form haemoglobin (the substance in red blood cells that carries oxygen around the blood). As such, it plays a vital role in good health, and it's important to know how much of it we should be consuming. Those who have a raised genetic requirement should consume more of it in food.

Vitamin B12 performs a similar function to vitamin B6 in that it helps to release energy from food, but also helps to make red blood cells and assists in the production of folic acid. It can be found in foods such as meat, salmon, cod, milk, cheese and eggs. Again, those who have a raised requirement should consume slightly more of these foods (proportionally of course).

Cruciferous vegetables

Cruciferous vegetables include broccoli, bok choy, cress, cauliflower, cabbage and kale, and should be consumed on a daily basis. They are classified in the Brassicaceae family and are a rich source of vitamins, fibre and phytochemicals. Again, they are easy to add into a smoothie (I use kale and cress quite frequently), as well as lightly steaming before adding to a main meal. They can help with the removal of toxins, and are very easy to source. Always go for organic and buy as

close to the source as possible. The DNA test can detect whether you
have a normal or raised requirement, to ensure you're getting what
you need from these vegetables.

Conclusion

The amount of information we can get from a DNA test will
continue to develop, but already there is a huge amount you can
learn from your DNA. Using this information will be key to
prolonging your healthspan, and ensuring we're getting you the
right amount of vitamins and minerals *based on your unique genotype*.
The recommended daily allowances are only a guideline, and if you
want to understand what you need, you'll need to dovetail the DNA
with expert guidance and support to optimise your health.

TOP TIP

Ever since I did a DNA test to understand what my dietary
requirements are for crucial vitamins and other health-related
factors, I've been starting the day with a vegetable and fruit
smoothie. The test results told me what my requirements
are for cruciferous vegetables, Omega 3, vitamin B6 and
anti-oxidants, and I now ensure I get a good proportion of my
daily needs in a morning smoothie. It's quick and easy to do,
and a great way to start the day. You'll need a liquid base
for the smoothie, and I use coconut milk. Coconuts are very
nutritious and rich in fibre, and vitamins C, E, B1, B3, B5 and
B6 as well as many minerals including selenium, calcium,
magnesium, sodium and phosphorus. This is also ideal if you
are lactose intolerant, as I am

Understanding how your body works

There are tests you can do to determine whether you have any food intolerances or if there are things going on in your gut which are impacting your ability to digest properly and process nutrients. If budget permits, it's advisable to do those tests and work out whether there's something that's not agreeing with you. Often it will be obvious because you'll notice side effects such as bloating, gas or gastrointestinal discomfort, but sometimes the symptoms can be hidden or harder to discern. The vitamin D3 test is one I always recommend to clients because it's so easy to do, and costs very little. The results are also very simple to interpret so do not require complex consultation fees.

Other tests that are useful are thyroid performance, basal body temperature and the adrenal stress test, all of which were discussed earlier on.

Supplementation

A key part of personalising your diet is understanding the role of supplementation. Always ask yourself the question, could I be getting this from food, and if so, try and include more of those foods in your diet. A supplement is just that, it's not a substitute. Of equal importance, if you have specific requirements for additional vitamins and minerals, go for a good quality supplement and definitely do not go for the cheapest brand. (I usually use a brand called Cytoplan.) Before making the decision to take a supplement, make sure you need to do so. It's become quite common practice to take a multivitamin, but many people I know buy a cheap brand and use it blindly, i.e. they haven't gone through a rigorous testing process to understand what their personal requirements are. Finding that out, and then finding out the right supplements for you is crucial.

Other considerations for personalising your nutrition

Listen to your body

I've said it before, but this is really important. A plan needs to be adapted and flexed according to how you feel, amongst other factors. Some of these factors might include:

- Stress levels

- Lifeload

- Activity levels

- Health

- Environment

- Hormonal changes

- Pregnancy

- Mood

Sometimes less is more; you may get more value from abandoning your planned exercise session and eating a good meal or watching a film instead. It's quite a skill learning how to interpret the signs your body sends you, but trust me, it rarely sends out false signals. It takes maturity to listen and respond, rather than blithely pressing on with the plan and potentially getting sick, injured, overtraining or losing interest because the enjoyment has gone.

Understand the restrictions of time and budget

There will be times when you don't have enough time to prepare the quality of meal you had planned for. Don't stress about this. Having the odd meal or day when it doesn't go to plan is OK. There are some fairly decent food preparation and delivery services available now (it's a growing market), which can help if you are time-poor or unused to cooking! The basic premise of these services is they source and prepare the ingredients for a meal, package them to keep things fresh and then delivery the box of uncooked ingredients to your door. All you have to do is cook them according to the instructions. The company I continually see is Hello Fresh! but other companies include Natoora, Marley Spoon and Gousto, with others popping up all the time.

Our philosophy is to encourage clients to cook fresh meals using ingredients that they've sourced and selected themselves. I'm always delighted if a client tells me they've been down to the local farmer's market and hand-picked the ingredients for the week's meals. When I got into nutrition four years ago, I signed up to a local vegetable scheme called Local Greens. They worked with farms within a 60-mile radius of London, and delivered whatever vegetables were ready to come out of the ground that week. You never knew what you were getting until the day before, but it was so fresh it was often still coated in soil. I often didn't even know what some of the vegetables were, and part of the fun was working out what they were (take a photo of it and send it to Mum), then working out what to do with them. We try to encourage clients to fall in love with food, and that includes sourcing, preparation and cooking. If you find it hard to fall in love with cooking, then at least learn to love the fact you're eating fresh foods cooked there and then, free from preservatives and excess sugar and salt.

Apps that track nutrition

There are now many different apps that help you to personalise what you're eating, and then track and monitor macronutrients and calories. The main player is MyFitnessPal, but others include Lose It, Noom Coach and FatSecret, amongst others. Many now include barcode scanners to help you easily record foods purchased in the supermarket, and are generally pretty accurate. It all helps to ensure you're following a plan, and technology is about to explode in the health, nutrition and fitness world, as I'll discuss next.

Chapter 6:
Wearable Technology

This is a huge growth area at the moment, and one that will have a major impact on the sports, health and fitness market in the UK and globally. The global market for wearable technology was recently estimated to be $2 billion, with one in six Americans wearing some form of wearable tech (according to a Nielsen report). Audit and accountancy firm PwC estimate that the connected health market will be worth $61 billion by 2020. Of respondents surveyed by PwC about this market, 40% said they believed tech increased the control their have over their health and fitness.

The market for wearable fitness tracking devices is big business, with the number of devices produced expected to increase from 17.7 million in 2014 to 40.7 million this year. According to research firm IDC, more than 100 million fitness devices that fit on your wrist like a watch will be sold across the globe by 2019. There will be 1.7 billion mobile health apps available by the end of 2017 (PwC), and the Health Secretary Jeremy Hunt has said he wants one quarter of all smartphone users accessing and updating their medical records by 2020. Even companies that you would not typically associate with technology are in on it; Tag Heuer have made a watch that tracks health-related data as part of their Connected range. US clothing giant Ralph Lauren have created a range of polo shirts that work with your iPhone or Apple Watch to deliver real-time data such as heart rate, breathing depth and balance, and other key metrics via a detachable Bluetooth-enabled box. Wearable technology or 'connected clothing' as it's also known, adds yet another layer to your ability to personalise your health and fitness.

Connected fitness

Wrist-based technology

What was once a market dominated by a handful of key players (Fitbit being the main one), there are now lots of established manufacturers and start-ups who've entered the sector looking to do something different or better. Cloudtag, Moov Now, Jawbone, Apple, Garmin, Misfit, Tom-Tom, MS Band and MyZone are just some of the better-known manufacturers all competing for market share. Most of them offer similar functionality; calories, steps, stairs, heart rate, sleep patterns, smart notifications and in some cases, caller ID. I used to wear a Fitbit Charge HR because I'd read some reviews and I thought at the time that it offered good value for money, and was reasonably reliable. Having reviewed the market as part of my research for this book (note I didn't get to actually trial any products, although that would have been a lot of fun), there is a lot of choice and they all broadly do the same thing, but there is currently some really innovative technology out there, which we're now including as part of our packages and wearing ourselves.

Wrist-based devices

Many of these devices do very similar things, and there are a number of them on the market, ranging from £65 to over £400. Almost all the wrist-based devices allow you to track the number of steps you've walked per day, and are usually pre-programmed to a target of 10,000 steps. This is a useful tool to have to keep track of your activity levels, although there is a degree of inaccuracy with most devices. I've noticed that some people treat the 10,000 steps as the daily target and once they've hit the target, feel they can eat with impunity. The 10,000 steps target is simply a guideline and should be considered the minimum that you do each day just to maintain base fitness. It's great if you've been very sedentary, but should not be the full extent of your daily efforts.

If you're wondering, the magic number of 10,000 is believed to have originated in the 1964 Tokyo Olympics, according to Catrine Tudor-Locke, an associate professor at the Pennington Biomedical Research Centre at Louisiana State University. Apparently in the run-up to the Olympics, the use of pedometers became very popular and a device was launched called the manpo-kei, which means 10,000 steps.

Most of these devices track the distance you've covered, the number of stairs climbed and the total number of calories burned (based on the personal information you enter when you set up the device). You can usually link to an app to record all your food and drink, which is really handy. It's surprising what you'll forget about your daily food and drink intake, but typing it into an app is a really good way of becoming more conscious about what you put into your body. Having an app to hand (such as the ones I mentioned in the previous chapter) means you can plan snacks and meals to ensure you're getting in enough calories or not over consuming them when on the move. This is particularly helpful when you've got specific fitness goals that depend on good nutrition delivered at the right times.

In summary, the market for wrist-based wearable technology is now more competitive, and you can get a reasonably reliable device for under £100 if you're willing to trade functionality for price. I definitely recommend using some form of wearable tech to help you personalise your workouts and nutrition plans, and monitor and track your data in real-time. Don't get too bent out of shape about accuracy though; most devices in this price range are inaccurate by up to 30%.

Case Study

Sam is a partner in a City law firm who works long hours, has a family at home and often skips meals. During the first consultation, we established that she often forgot to eat (probably a result of adrenalin caused by stress), and when things quietened down, hunger would hit her and she'd go for the first thing she could find – usually refined carbohydrates like biscuits, cakes or pastries. She was concerned about the number of calories she was taking in. I was concerned at the nutritional quality of the calories. We agreed she would wear a device to record her activity levels, and record her food in the app. As a result, she was able to appreciate the number of calories she was taking in from so little food, and how long the gaps were between her meals. She now eats regularly from foods which are simple, but high in nutritional value.

Fingerwear

It is now possible to get information such as body temperature, motion, sleep and heart rate on a ring, worn on the finger. A Finnish company called Ōura has developed a ring which they are calling smart jewelry, and it is arguably a lot more stylish than a wrist- based device. As soon as I heard about this technology, I've been wearing it. It's similar in size and appearance to a signet ring, and available in black or white, and it's the world's first ring-sized wellness computer. It has all the standard functionality of most wearable tech devices but it is the most accurate sleep tracker on the market, and offers intelligent analysis of your data, making it ideal for those people who want really tailored advice. I'll talk more about the ring at the end of this chapter.

Footwear

There are a few companies who have launched wearable technology inside a sock or a shoe sole. TRAXXs is a French company whose XSole is on the market. It's a device that fits into the sole of your shoe and measures your speed, distance covered, intensity and the number of calories burned. The manufacturer's claim on their website is that it can also be used for tracking people, such as a caregiver who might be able to use it to keep an eye on an elderly relative's movements.

Another player in the market is Arion, manufactured by a company called ATO-gear, who have a sole with six in-shoe sensors which respond with data about running gait, according to where pressure is on the foot.

Sensoria have created a sock which transmits data about the cadence, speed, distance and technique of the wearer. I talked to a representative from Sensoria whilst researching this book, and I've included a summary later in the chapter.

Bodywear

During my research, I came across a company called OMSignal (who partnered with Ralph Lauren on their wearables range). OMSignal manufacturer a sports bra called OMbra which has built-in technology to track heart rate, distance travelled and calories expended, but also data about your breathing including rhythm, fatigue levels and biometric effort. The data is downloaded to an app and helps you to understand where you're wasting energy and how you can exercise more efficiently. Advances in technology have done away with the need for a strap to monitor heart rate as it's all built into the bra.

Several companies manufacture t-shirts and vests with technology built-in to monitor heart rate and other data. Another interesting find is the Spartan Boxer Brief, which has been designed to protect male genitalia from the cellular damage caused by mobile phones and Wi-Fi radiation. Spartan have interwoven pure silver fibres into their cotton weave, creating a high-tech fabric that shields against the electromagnetic effect of mobile phones and Wi-Fi signals. The fabric is designed to protect the genitals from potential sperm damage caused by radiation with the aim of preserving fertility.

Taking wearable technology to another level is a device called Thync, which has been recently developed to help users feel more awake and alert, or more calm, depending on what the sensors are picking up. The unit itself is fitted on the side of the forehead and connects to your smartphone using Bluetooth technology. The device sends minor electrical signals through the skin to muscles of the face and neck, whilst stimulating certain areas of the brain to create desired response.

Whatever you might think about wearable technology, it's a big market, driving a lot of innovation and attracting a lot of investment. High-street giant Top Shop have created an innovation programme to help discover start-ups in the wearable tech space, and they've stated that one of their goals is to be a leading provider of wearable tech at an affordable price point. An increasing number of jewelry companies are striving to create products at the intersection of fashion and technology, and the connected clothing market continues to grow and be the centre of innovation. Apple, often the leaders in this space, are very close to developing a workable device worn on your wrist which no longer needs your smartphone to be close by in order to download data. It's a very exciting space and those in my industry who don't embrace it will get left behind.

The advantages of wearable technology

So what are the advantages of wearable tech for the everyday person who wants to personalise their health and fitness, without spending a fortune? Here's why I think wearable tech can help with the personalisation of exercise:

- Encourages personal responsibility and self-monitoring

- Helps to create an awareness of how active you are (or are not)

- Helps you monitor your heart rate and training zones

- Creates an environment where you can compete online with others

- Provides access to data that can help you identify when to step up or step down your training based on how you are feeling (intelligent training)

- Allows you to approximate your calorie intake each day to better plan your meals and snacks

- Provides a one-stop-shop for most of the health and fitness-related data that recreational athletes require to stay healthy and active

Since I started using wearable tech a while ago, I've become much more aware of how much I'm moving. It's actually been quite eye-opening; there are days when I think I've been quite active, but in fact I've only done approximately half my target of 5,000 steps, which is some way off the target programmed into the device and the amount recommended by the UK National Obesity Forum (10,000 steps). I am a very fit and active person, but I will confess the device is having a positive effect on my activity levels too. I also find it very useful for tracking my sleep, which often falls short of the eight-hour target. The benefits of the device will be much more stark and game-changing for those who are less active though. If you already do several hours of exercise a week, walking a few extra thousand steps per day is not going to be hugely significant (although certainly not to be sniffed at). For people who are more sedentary though, the results could be truly life-changing.

Are there downsides?

I don't think there are many downsides to wearable tech. One major manufacturer did have to recall one of its models due to skin problems caused by the device, but this has since been rectified. If you are the type of person who over-obsesses with such devices, and becomes fixated with the stats (have you ever seen a runner fall off a curb or run into a lamppost because they're constantly looking at their watch?), then perhaps you should be careful with it. My clients report that they find the calorie monitoring and food logging very useful, but personally and professionally I am not a fan of calorie-counting per se, so for someone who has issues with food this might not be a positive feature for them. It's also important to allow for slight inaccuracies of data in some devices, as I mentioned earlier. If the device is 200 calories per day inaccurate either way, that could add up to quite a significant calorie increase or deficit, depending on your goals. I think a healthy way to view it is as another tool you can use for personalisation, and not the be-all-and-end-all.

Personalising your sleep

Understanding how your lifestyle affects your sleep, which in turn affects your daily performance, is crucial to staying healthy and having the energy to enjoy our daily activities. The best way to figure out what's going on when you sleep is to wear a sleep tracker, or use your smartphone. The advantage of using your smartphone is it's there already, at no extra expense. The disadvantage is the potential inaccuracy. You can also use some of the wrist-based wearables, but personally I use the ŌURAring to monitor my sleep. The ŌURAring is the most accurate sleep tracker on the market, and the whole premise of the device is built around sleep, not activity *per se*. The ŌURAring tracks your sleep using respiratory rate, movement, heart rate, pulse waves and body temperature. The ring itself sits on any finger of either hand, is comfortable and stylish, and crucially is highly accurate. The inside of the ring contains sensors that are continuously collecting data whilst you sleep, and then feeding that data back to you via the app. The app gives you a headline number, which is your sleep score, determined by a number of contributors including sleep timing (how well attuned you are to your circadian rhythms), sleep efficiency (percentage of time you spend asleep after going to bed), disturbances (caused by waking or getting up in the night), REM sleep (rapid eye movement, i.e. when dreaming or falling asleep), sleep latency (the time it takes to fall asleep), deep sleep (the most restorative sleep you can get), total sleep, and your resting heart rate (RHR, the number of times your heart beats per minute when at rest). RHR is very interesting because it's a good measurement of sleep quality, as well as overall health. A high RHR compared to normal is a good indicator of how stressed you are or whether you are getting sick. An exceptionally high or low RHR can also indicate a sign of increased need for recovery. The human body is very good at giving out signals to indicate its state of wellness, and the ŌURAring amplifies those signals and makes them visible via the data on the app.

Collecting this data via the ŌURA app is a useful way to track your sleep. I work with clients who tell me they get eight or nine hours sleep, yet often wake feeling tired and unrestored. Analysing their ŌURA data can be very telling; despite going to bed early, they sleep lightly, getting very little deep sleep and wake frequently. Having access to this data means we can look at lifestyle modifications that can help improve their sleep scores. Examples of this include working out earlier in the day, having a good pre-bedtime ritual (I've started meditating for five or ten minutes before bed and it's really helped), avoiding caffeine, avoiding overstimulating the brain with screens or television an hour before bedtime, eating earlier in the evening, or reading a fictional book rather than a business book or something mentally taxing.

You can personalise your sleep and retune your circadian rhythms by modifying your bedroom. I use blackout blinds, and have low lighting in the bedroom. You can buy low blue light bulbs which filter out the blue light emitted by conventional light bulbs, and don't disturb your melatonin production. (Melatonin is the hormone produced by the pineal gland and regulates our sleep cycles, so if this is disturbed, for example by the lights by your bed, then it can affect your sleep). Having a mattress made from organic materials and customised for your body (for example a memory mattress) and good quality pillows is helpful, and a sprinkle of lavender oil on the pillow at night can be very calming. If you are someone that struggles to relax before bed, try introducing this little tip into your bedtime routine: make a list of what you've achieved that day, and then another list of what needs to be done the following day. I've found this is really helpful in valuing that day's output, and brain-dumping everything I didn't get done but will prioritise for tomorrow. It means I can go to bed with a clear head.

Personalised medicine

It won't be long before personalised medicine follows wearable tech; it's already there for those who can afford it. It's likely that in future, insurance companies will issue these devices to help track patient health, and offer lower premiums to those who meet their targets. (Several insurance companies are already doing this by offering clients the opportunity to install a box in the car that monitors how they're driving.) Of course there is the thorny issue of privacy to be considered, which will put many people off, and some might not want their insurance company to have such detailed information about their health, lifestyle choices, dietary habits and exercise levels.

Personalised medicine is available for the very wealthy, but for most of us, the one-size-fits-all approach to medication still applies, and we find solutions to our medical problems through a combination of expert guidance and trial and error. It is my belief that devices that enable us to self-monitor our performance levels will help us to take more personal responsibility for our health and wellbeing, which can only be a good thing for us, the NHS, and all other government-subsidised healthcare around the world. Of course, you can use your smartphone to track this data, although you'll lose out on some of the personal data such as heart rate. If that's not so important to you though, most smartphones will collect data such as steps, calorie estimates, etc., and will suffice if you don't want to invest in a wearable device.

Case Study

Jay is a 29-year old entrepreneur from Birmingham. His business specialises in helping primary schools develop high performing cultures. Before Jay started his business, he worked at a large corporate in the mobile technology sector, where he became disenfranchised with the work and eventually burned out. During this time, he was regularly exercising, but following a certain type of training that had been recommended by a trainer who had got results through those methods. The training was high intensity and very cardio-based, and for a while this worked for him, and he enjoyed it. After a while though, the lack of personalisation started to show. The workouts that were being prescribed to him by a trainer became less enjoyable, and he started to feel awful. The diet was very protein heavy, with lots of meat, which he found indigestible and made him slow and sluggish. Despite his nutrition programme containing the industry prescribed balance of micro and macronutrients, it wasn't working for him. He also suspected that the protein shakes, full of whey, were hard for his body to process, and that he might be intolerant to lactose. Frustrated and feeling wrecked, Jay ditched the previous training programme and nutrition plan and started working out on his own, using an app called Stronglifts 5x5 (www.stronglifts.com/5x5) on his smartphone to create an exercise programme. The app automatically periodised the workouts (increased the weight or reps according to how many workouts had been completed). He also moved in with his girlfriend who is Japanese, and he immediately noticed the benefits of eating a cleaner diet with more carbohydrates and oily fish. He lost weight, regained his muscle mass and his body found its natural set point. He has also used an app called HabitBull (www.habitbull.com) to help establish a good pattern of exercise and to give up sugar (which he had tried a few times before, but having an app to check on his success each day made it easy for him to keep up the willpower through the cravings). He used another app called Sleep Cycle to help him to track his sleep, and he found he was able to get to bed earlier, sleep longer and more deeply. In doing all this, Jay has personalised all the important aspects of his life using his instinct and a process of trial and error. This takes time and patience, and can be very frustrating, but I'm sure that Jay would say it was all worth it in the end. He says: "I no longer feel like fitness is a hobby or chore because personalisation has made it part of my life. I no longer consciously think about my diet as I've found what is right for me, and this has all led to improving my own body confidence and putting me in the best shape I have been for years."

The future of wearable tech for health, fitness and nutrition

I interviewed some of the companies mentioned in this book to find out who they thought their product was for, what needs it met and what they thought the future of wearable tech looked like. Here are their responses.

Sharlene Sternberg of Sensoria Inc.

Senoria Inc. is an American company based in Redmond, Washington. According to their website, the company "designs, develops and produces body-sensing smart garments as truly wearable devices that make meaningful impact." The company was founded by three

Microsoft executives who spotted an opportunity to bring wearable tech to the fitness market. They launched their first product, the Sensoria Sock, in 2014, and have now developed a sports bra and t-shirt range aimed at consumers. Their strapline is "The Garment is the Computer®."

I spoke to Sharlene to find out what defines their products, what need they're meeting and what Sensoria think the future of wearable technology is. As I anticipated, the drive behind these products for the fitness market is personalisation. The founders and developers recognise that everyone from the recreational runner to professional athlete is looking for ways to monitor, track and ultimately improve their performance using data they can glean from testing or technology. Their flagship product, the Smart Sock, contains sensors on three parts of the foot which report on things like cadence, speed, pace, calories as well as technique, feeding that data back to an app via Bluetooth wireless technology. The app can be monitored by a coach or by the user themselves. It's the same principle for the sports bra and the t-shirt.

Interestingly, Sensoria have identified another market for this type of technology, which is healthcare. They have partnerships with a handful of healthcare companies to provide technology that helps with the treatment of diabetic feet, with the fitting of prosthetics, fall detection and rehabilitation. Insurance companies are now getting wise to the technology, and we may well see a future where insurance policies are discounted for those who agree to use wearable tech that can be monitored remotely.

Future developments will see Sensoria launching smaller, embeddable products that can be fitted to clothing or body parts, but perform the same functions as the wearable tech kit. Sternberg thinks this is the next step for this type of technology, and the company are about to launch a version of their products which removes the need for you to have your smartphone with you – you can sync to your smartphone once the run or exercise session is finished via Bluetooth. I asked Sternberg whether she thought there were any downsides to wearable tech, and aside from accuracy (which everyone is working on improving), she struggled to think of anything. I am inclined to agree.

Petteri Lahtela of ŌURA

ŌURA is a Finnish company based in the city of Oulu in northern Finland. Oulu is renowned as a technology hub for medical and health technology, and is the home of company Polar Electro, who launched the world's first heart rate monitors, and is also the home of mobile phone giant Nokia. Some of Nokia's most significantly and market-breaking inventions were created in Oulu. CEO and Co-founder of ŌURA, Petteri Lahtela says, "We (Oulu) have a lot of that heritage of creating high-end consumer products to global markets". One of the founding principles behind their products is a desire to help others to enable, reach and then maintain their human potential, which is my purpose, professionally and personally.

I found my conversation with Petteri Lahtela fascinating. There are many parallels between their company's ethos and mine, despite the technical difference in our products and services. One of the founding principles behind their products is a desire to help others to enable, reach and then maintain their human potential, which is my purpose, professionally and personally. Lahtela believes that diseases and fatigue are a result of imbalances in the body's systems, often caused by the presence, or lack of, stress, inflammation, diet and exercise. He believes that technology could be used to track and monitor this vital data to develop a holistic picture of the daily mental and physical load being carried by a person. (I talk a lot about allostatic load and lifeload in my first book, *Rise and Shine: Recover from burnout and get back to your best.*)

The ŌURA ring

The device itself is a ring that sits snugly on any finger on either hand, and can be worn 24/7. It also happens to be a computer with a Bluetooth connection that allows for easy download and automatic updates. It's durable, scratch resistant, waterproof, and has a timeless design. At the time of writing the retail price starts from EUR 329.00, making it affordable for many, and by no means the most expensive device on the market. It has been extensively tested by research groups at highly prestigious American universities, and this research supports their claim that it is the most reliable sleep measurement device on the market. One of the target audiences is executives and entrepreneurs who have a very *stressful life, or struggle with their work/life balance and want a personalised solution to help them self-monitor meaningful data points such as sleep quality and recovery from daily mental and physical load in relation to activity levels, daily lifestyle choices and rhythms.*

How is it different from wrist-based tech?

Where the ŌURA ring differs is that it's an intelligent device that measures how your body responds to your activities and daily movement, and helps the user to identify how those things affect sleep quality. It also provides the ideal daily activity target based on how much quality sleep you've got. Lahtela says "the ŌURA ring provides personalised, actionable insights to the user to help them make better choices based on how well they have recovered and recharged". Where other devices are about getting you to move more, the ŌURA ring intelligently analyses your data and determines what you should be doing and how hard you should be pushing. It works by tracking the physiological responses of your body whilst you sleep, measuring your pulse waveform and heart rate dynamics, body temperature, and movement with what the company calls "research-level accuracy."

Intelligent analysis

For many entrepreneurs and executives, pushing hard when they should be slowing down is not a problem; that's their current mindset and is why they're burning out. This intelligent device will be able to understand and interpret your daily load, and then respond and advise the user accordingly. The beauty of this technology is that's it's still early days for the developers; the future for the ŌURA ring will be based on adding benefits, integrating with daily routines and adding more benefits to help improve the wearer's cognitive and physical performance by cross-correlating between the various data points.

The (wearable tech) world according to Lahtela

I asked Lahtela what he thought the future held for the wearable tech industry. He said he thought technology would become even more personalised, and allow for more intelligent analysis. Lahtela believes that awareness of the importance of sleep and recovery is the next big wave, not only in wearables but in health and wellness market in general. "Understanding the restorative nature of sleep is essential since that's the only way to find ways to improve the recovery from daily mental and physical load." He foresees a future where devices would work alongside other providers such as insurance companies, healthcare providers and caregivers to supply information that can help reduce the rate of chronic diseases, and help to manage diseases once they've manifested themselves. He also thought wearable tech would start working alongside genetics and epigenetics to provide a more holistic view of a person, which I think is a very exciting future for all of us.

Personally, I love the ŌURA ring. I've bought one and will be wearing it night and day to monitor my sleep and energy levels, particularly given I've suffered from burnout in 2012, and am understandably cautious to ensure this doesn't happen again. The intelligence interpretation of data is what really appeals to me; it's not about setting targets like 10,000 steps (although for many people, this is a really important feature and they do need to move more), but about listening to your body and understanding the physical and emotional life load that you're carrying, and how you can recover from that load. If you're sleep hasn't been restorative, then the device might advise you to take it easy that day, maybe aim for 6,000 steps but taken as part of a gentle walk, preferably somewhere quiet and amongst nature. I've worked with clients who are incredibly frustrated because they are getting to bed early and spending up to eight or nine hours in bed, but waking up feeling exhausted, and they can't understand why. There's a huge difference between the amount of time you spend in bed and the amount and quality of REM or deep sleep that you enjoy. Now, link this data to a nutrition plan and an overall holistic therapeutic plan, and you have something very valuable that sits at the intersection between technology and personalised health.

Bodyscanning

Another way to personalise your workouts is to understand exactly what's going on in the inside of your body as well as what's visible from the outside. This isn't super-new technology, but you can have scans to determine information such as:

- Bone mineral density

- Total muscle mass

- Total fat mass

- Muscle imbalances

- Total body fat percentage

- Visceral fat percentage (fat around your vital organs)

The scans are called DEXA scans, and a simple Google search will find several results of companies who offer the service. The scans are not very expensive – typically between £150 to £500 – but can reveal significantly important information about what's happening inside your body. It's quite possible to be lean and fit, yet still have a lot of fat around the vital organs inside your body. It's also a useful test if you're an older female (pre- menopausal), because it will ascertain your bone density, which is an important signifier of your risk of osteopenia and osteoporosis. (Osteoporosis occurs typically in post- menopausal women, as the menopause results in a significant drop in estrogen levels which affect bone density. This can be countered by resistance-exercises such as moderate weight lifting, body weight exercises and running. Osteopenia is the precursor to osteoporosis).

DEXA scanning is safe, and takes about five minutes to do. You lie still on a bed whilst a mechanical arms passes over your body, feeding the results back to a computer. The amount of radiation emitted is the equivalent to eating a small bag of Brazil nuts, so there's no risk of excess radiation to worry about. That said, you should avoid having the test done if you are pregnant. I believe this data is very useful as a way of benchmarking where you're at now with your health. It provides you with a clear picture of how your body looks from the inside, as well as fitness tests that can determine your physical fitness. You can use this data along with the DNA results to plan your workouts, but perhaps more importantly, to create a bespoke diet and nutrition plan.

Case Study

Meg is a 38-year old lawyer living in London. We've been working with her for over two years. Prior to joining us, Meg had a DEXA body scan to understand what her total body fat percentage was and how much visceral fat she had inside her. When I met Meg, she appeared quite lean. She was 5' 10" tall, and a size 12. We went through her current state of fitness and performed some basic fitness tests, and she performed reasonably well for someone who had been away from regular exercise for a while. We talked about nutrition, and I could see there were several areas we could work on but it didn't sound too bad. Looking at the DEXA results, I was shocked. She actually had a high body fat percentage (30%, which is the border of overweight and obese), and a lot of visceral fat and fat around her gluteal-femoral region (upper thighs and stomach). It was a perfect illustration of the fact that all is not what it seems from the outside. We used this data alongside the DNA test to create a bespoke diet and exercise plan that targeted this 'problem fat'. The plan worked; Meg reduced her body fat by between 0.5 – 1% each week and gained up to 1lb of muscle every four weeks, which was excellent in terms of her overall health and what was practical and manageable.

The Naked Fit Scanner

The Naked Fit Scanner is the world's first 3D body scanner. It's a full length mirror which connects to a turntable that you stand on. 20 seconds later it's rotated you 360 degrees and scanned your body. Naked captures your 3D body model and then sends the images to an app on your smartphone. You can set up two images of your body taken at monthly intervals for instance, and scroll across them to get comparative data on body composition changes like fat loss and muscle gain. Whereas previously these kinds of measurements were unavailable or done manually (which is very susceptible to human error), now the scans can be done in real-time. It's another exciting new technological development, and can be used at home as well as in gyms. Needless to say we've ordered one. The only downside is they don't ship until March 2017.

Chapter 7:
Personalising your mindset

Let's recap on what we've discussed so far. We've talked about how we can use cutting-edge technology such as DNA testing to personalise what we do. The third and fifth chapters focused on using that technology specifically for nutrition and fitness, with examples of how people have used that information to get to their goals quicker and more efficiently. There is a world of difference though between knowing this information, and applying it. That difference is attitude and mindset.

Michael Serwa

Michael Serwa is a life coach based in London. He works with the elite using his signature 'no bullshit' approach. He's a 33-year old who in just five years has ensured he is now one of the UK's highest-paid life coaches. Michael and I met as we are both part of a network called Key People of Influence (KPI) in London. He is now a friend and a client, and his story is quite remarkable.

Michael is from Poland, born to parents who, in his words, "were average." They were a good, loving family but they were not entrepreneurs or business owners and had no access to any personal wealth or money. They hadn't achieved anything spectacular. Michael was himself very average at school, and didn't excel at any particular subject or stand out academically. What Michael did possess though was a desire to pursue greatness. He felt there was something out there for him, if he put himself in the right environment to make it happen. Keen to find his purpose, he came to London in 2005, hungry for success.

Hungry in other ways as well, as he was penniless. He travelled from Poland to London via bus, because it was the cheapest way. It took 27 hours to make the journey, but he had spent all his money on the ticket because he felt that if he was to be successful, he had to be in a huge, thriving economy like London. When he arrived, he spent the first two weeks living in a squat whilst he found some basic accommodation, and bought food from a low-cost supermarket using money lent by friends. He told me he had a major bust-up with his girlfriend one day because she wanted to buy grapes, which he felt were a luxury they could not afford. Every penny was made to work as hard as it could and there was no unnecessary expenditure. Shortly after moving to London, he began his first career in fashion retail. Then, six years later, he set up his coaching business. Everyone around him thought he was mad. 'Why set up a business where there's so much competition?' was the standard response. Michael started by charging £20/hour for his services, and he worked solidly for two and a half years, never taking a holiday or even a day off. As he picked up clients, he started charging more. £50/hour, then £75/hour, until he had built up a business and a reputation that enabled him to set his own prices. A client today might pay up to £20,000 a year for his services, and he has a waiting list of people looking to work with him. So how did he do it? I spent some time talking to Michael about what makes one person successful over another, and what his definition is of a winner's mindset.

A winning mindset

Firstly, Michael believes you are not born with a winning or a losing mindset. It's not in your genes. A mindset is created by you and the way you choose to think about things, as well as the environment you're in and all your experiences. He believes that the right mindset combined with three other elements are the ingredients to success of any kind.

The three other elements are:

- Passion

- Hustle

- Persistence

Passion

We hear a lot about how passionate people are about something – watch any TV talent contest whether it's Dragons Den or X Factor and all you'll hear about is how passionate the contestants are, and how much they want something. Passion isn't about how much you want something, it's about how much you believe something lines up with your values. Then you can claim you're passionate about it, that you believe in it and enjoy it, whatever that thing is. For Michael, that was life coaching. He felt with every fibre of his being that life coaching was what he was put here to do. And that's one reason why he has been able to build such a reputation for himself by helping over 400 clients over the last five years. But here's the rub: passion on its own is not enough. It's important, sure, but you also need another important factor: hustle.

Hustle

Hustle is basically working hard, but Michael believes that hard work only makes sense when it is executed intelligently. It's not working hard - it's working smart at working hard. Lots of people work hard, yet have very little. In fact, most of the UK economy is fuelled by hard-working people who in reality have very little disposable income or wealth. Someone with hustle is someone who has a clear idea of what their goals are, and how they're going to get to them. It's not working hard, it's working smart. Hustlers will keep themselves fit by toning their bodily muscles, and they'll also be training their 'hustle muscle' every day by following some of the other principles described in this chapter. Personally, I hustle every day to win another client, court another potential partner, create another PR opportunity, put out another great piece of content and make clients, partners and my team happy.

Persistence

The other thing you will need to be successful is persistence. Let's look at Michael's example again. He came to London with nothing, then after setting up his coaching business he worked for two and a half years without a single day off. How was he able to do this? Because he had passion; he had hustle (loads of it), and he was persistent. He knew that he would get to his goal of being the highest paid life coach in the UK. He knew it wouldn't happen quickly, but every day he got a little closer to his goal. He was patient.

When you start with a winning mindset and you add passion, hustle and persistence to the mix, that's when the success will happen.

What drives a winning mindset?

There are other factors that we can consider that create a winning mindset. The first is general attitude. Now you're reading this book, so you're probably not the average person. You've identified with the concept of personalisation, and you've probably already invested time and money into your health, nutrition and fitness plans. You bought this book because you wanted to understand how you can improve yourself in the most time-efficient and effective way. In purchasing and making time to read this book, you've just demonstrated to yourself that you have passion, hustle and persistence. Here are the other important factors to consider:

Environment

This is probably the most important of all. Your environment will drive your performance levels, it's as simple as that. In 2015, I went on a 40-week brand accelerator programme called Key Person of Influence. The programme helps business leaders and entrepreneurs to transform their businesses by focusing on five areas: Pitch, Publish, Products, Profile and Partnerships. I learnt a lot on the programme (going on the programme was one of the best business decisions I've ever made), but my personal performance levels went through the roof because I was taken into an environment where I was surrounded by entrepreneurs or well-known business leaders talking about how they solve meaningful problems. We met regularly outside of the programme (and still do), and continue to go to events where performance levels are high. Partnerships are formed, clients are introduced and ideas are swapped. Never underestimate the power of environment for driving performance.

Relationships

Look around at who you associate with. Are they high-performing people? Look amongst your friends, work colleagues, your partner and even family. Is there someone there who is a toxic influence? Someone who is very negative or has a closed-mindset? These people are unhealthy to be around and will affect your performance.

Get rid of them. It's up to you to remove yourself from them; you are personally responsible for who you spend time with. If your goals are to get fitter, spend time with people who are as motivated as you are to get fitter, and people who have the fitness you want to emulate. If you want to lose weight, hire a fitness coach who has lost weight and mix with people who have achieved significant weight loss. Surround yourself with people who have the mindset (and therefore the life) you want.

Strategy

This links back to hustle. Hard work isn't enough, there needs to be a strategy behind it. Having a really big goal (I've heard them described in business as BHAGs: Big Hairy Audacious Goals) is important, but you have to be patient. An entrepreneur I follow, Gary Vaynerchuk, has a big, hairy, audacious goal; he wants to buy the New York Jets someday. Maybe he will. Of course, Gary understands that is a big goal, but he is confidently going about his business and patiently building his wealth until such time as he can fulfill his boyhood dream. Set a big goal, then map your path to that goal by setting small targets which eventually add up to the big result. As you achieve these little wins, celebrate them, then move on to the next milestone. People who have a winning mindset will feed off results, and if they don't see them, will become frustrated. So, map your way to your ultimate goal, celebrate along the way, be persistent and never stop hustling.

Asking for help

Your general attitude is how you think, what you say to yourself and others, and how you behave. It's about self-respect, and therefore the level of respect you have for others. As I said, you probably already have a good general attitude, but many of us are unaware of how we sabotage ourselves with negative thoughts and that's why it's always good to work with a coach, whether it's a fitness coach, health coach or a life coach. As a business, we partner with all three to provide our clients with the support they need to get to their goals. Coaching can progress you far quicker than you could do on your own, and that's why elite athletes and businesspeople will have a coach on their team, even when they're at the top of their game. A person with a good attitude will know that there are no shortcuts, and won't be frustrated by this (persistence). A person with a winning mindset isn't afraid to ask for help, because they don't allow ego to get in the way. I used to take pride in creating and building things myself, without asking for help. I now see that this was misguided, and that the clever money is in asking for help and learning from others. All the people I have as role models now are coached by at least one person in their business and personal lives, and wouldn't be without them.

Here's a summary of what you need to have a winning mindset:

- Passion, hustle and persistence

- No limiting beliefs

- Positive thinking

- Ability to get resourceful

- Winning environment

- Positive role models

- Willingness to take risks

- Internal locus of control

- Find your voice

My seven guiding principles for optimising success

Manage your stress

We all suffer from stress at work from time to time, but for some people this can become very disabling, and start to affect how they feel about themselves and their career. Given that we spend a lot of time in the office or performing work functions, it's important to make sure that what you're doing isn't making you really unhappy, at least not for a prolonged period of time. Stress at work can affect life at home as well, and snowball into something more serious if not recognised and addressed.

Find your authenticity

Make sure what you do is an authentic expression of self – if you're doing something you really love, you will feel confident about it. Doing a job that isn't really you, but pays well will make you unhappy in the long run, and can lead to stress and burnout. If you're in a job because you thought it's what you should do, but would much rather be doing something else, this will take its toll. Consider what's really important to you, and do your best to find a job and a career that allows you to fulfil those aspirations. It's much more doable than you might think.

Setting boundaries

Identify and clearly delineate boundaries with regard to work, and make sure you respect them – if you do, it's easier to ask others to. Feeling stressed at work can be a result of doing too much, and then doing it badly. If you set rules around working hours, checking emails after hours, and what you are prepared to do above and beyond your defined role, then you'll feel more in control and be able to perform better as a result.

Focus on your fitness

Get physically fit (warning: this one's a biggie). Being physically fit means being mentally fit, and I really do believe the two are mutually inclusive. Start exercising, either with a trainer, partner or on your own if you're sufficiently self-motivated, and set aside a minimum of two sessions per week to exercise. Try and walk where possible, avoid escalators and lifts, and avoid sitting at your desk for more than 45 minutes without getting up and walking around a bit. (Tip: have a small tumbler of water on your desk so that you have to get up and refill the glass every so often)

Value your friends

Have a social life and friends who challenge you – this helps maintain perspective. Friends can challenge your thinking about situations at work, and can perhaps raise a flag when they see you getting stressed or your confidence dipping. A good friend can help you understand what you can do to improve your situation, and support you through difficult times.

Food and mood

Eat well – the connection between food and mood is very powerful – food and drink can make a profound difference to how you feel. Make sure you're eating regular meals, have some healthy snacks at your desk to maintain consistent blood sugar levels, and avoid sugar, caffeine and excess alcohol. Above all, eat a diet rich in vegetables and fruits, and drink plenty of water.

Beware overthinking!

Beware of paralysis by analysis! Don't overthink. A lot of stress comes from legitimately stressful situations, but a lot of it also comes from ourselves and how we think about things. Overthinking can be a dangerous thing, so try and deal with something once and then put it aside. Talking to a friend or partner can be really helpful in not overthinking a situation. Always try and get an outside perspective where you can.

Managing mobile devices

Set rules for your smart phone or Blackberry, especially at weekends and outside of working hours. We now live in a 24/7 culture, where we are accessible via email from almost every part of the world. There are very few places where you are not connected. It's up to you to manage that. Turn your phone off after 8pm, and let your colleagues know that you have a policy regarding phone use after hours. This sets the right level of expectation. Email can dominate our working day so having policies around email is also very effective at minimising stress. Take control of your day by deciding what your workload will be, as opposed to being to dictated by emails.

Chapter 8:
My Case Study

Background

I'm a 41-year old, who has worked in the City for most of my career. In 2012, I left my City career suffering from burnout. I took some time out and then retrained as a fitness coach and set up my company, Bodyshot. At the same time, I made some lifestyle changes; I started to eat very healthily and gave up alcohol completely. I exercised more frequently, and certainly more intelligently, and took a much greater interest in managing stress by using nutrition, sleep, relaxation techniques and slowing down a bit. Today, my working life is mainly spent outside or from time to time, inside at a desk, and I would describe my diet as healthy. I exercise for over an hour a day on average, and partake in a range of activities including boxing, circuit training, running, tennis and yoga on a weekly basis. I considered I ate fairly regularly, although my diet contained a lot of carbohydrates, which I thought I needed as I was doing a lot of exercise and being very physically active. Despite this, I found I was having some health issues that were starting to get in the way of life.

Medical overview

Fit and healthy, no medications, no injuries – only a recent diagnosis of asthma, which I was unsure about, and acid reflux for which I had been on a 4-week course of tablets.

The issues

There were four problems I wanted to understand and resolve. The first was my sugar addiction; I was eating two chocolate bars a day and could easily destroy a large bar of Cadbury's Whole Nut in one sitting, without sharing any of it. I would frequently crave chocolate, granola, biscuits, cakes, tarts… in fact anything sugary. Excuse the pun, but this was starting to eat at me.

The second problem was reflux and belching, especially after carbohydrates. Pizza would be the worst. At this point I hadn't directly connected the reflux or belching to anything else but had noticed the strong link to carbs.

The third problem was around sleep: I tended to fall asleep fairly quickly but would often wake around 4.45am or 5.15am – usually very close to those specific times. Once awake, I would feel hyper-alert, but I would force myself to stay in bed and would then eventually fall back to sleep. When I woke up again, I'd feel groggy and more tired than I did when I first woke.

The fourth problem was energy levels and a strange malaise that came over me overnight, and without any warning. The first episode of what I call my mystery sickness happened in September 2015. I woke up one Monday morning and immediately felt ill. My legs ached a lot, my stomach was knotted and I felt extremely lethargic – even without attempting to get up. When I did get out of bed, I had to descend the stairs using my bottom, and was then dry retching into the toilet. This lasted two days, during which I slept a lot and ate very little, drinking only herbal teas and water. On the third day I was able to go out, but was very weak and had to sit down frequently. This happened again, but to a slightly lesser extent in early December, around two months later. I had to cancel all my appointments and stay in bed until it passed. The main sensations were apathy and lethargy, knotted stomach and very achy legs. Just under two months later in February, it happened again, with very similar symptoms. It's hard to recall if there are any similarities in the circumstances around each sickness, but I think each coincided with consuming a large amount of lactose, and feeling quite tired and run down. At that time, I was doing more exercise than I do now.

What happened?

Concerned that this was becoming a regular occurrence, I went to the doctor and had a blood test. The results came back as normal with the exception of ferritin (iron), which was quite low. I wanted to take things a step further so I sat down with my genetic nutritionist and went through the series of tests that we now frequently offer to our clients. The tests included the DNA test (which I had taken in 2015), vitamin D3 and the adrenal stress test. I also recorded my basal body temperature for 10 consecutive days.

The results

DNA results

We reviewed the DNA results first. The headlines were that I have a very high sensitivity to carbohydrates, which means I process carbs very quickly and have a greater likelihood of storing them as fat. This will have a big impact on my blood sugar levels, and weight management. We thought it could also have a strong bearing on some of my digestive symptoms.

I also have a medium sensitivity to saturated fat, so I need to restrict the amount of daily saturated fat that I consume to a minimum (the recommended daily allowance at most). This sensitivity to both carbohydrates and saturated fat is quite an unusual combination, and one which we don't see very often, and would pose a slight challenge when it came to designing my food plan. The reports also told me I am intolerant to lactose, so I should avoid consuming all dairy products that contain lactose.

I am not intolerant to gluten, and therefore my risk of Coeliac Disease is very minimal, but cannot be ruled out. I have a raised sensitivity to salt and alcohol, but I am a slow metaboliser of caffeine, so it's advisory to have only two cups per day maximum, and nothing after midday (I drink decaf anyway).

The reports tell me I have a raised requirement for vitamin D3, anti-oxidants, cruciferous vegetables and omega 3s, but a normal requirement for vitamins B6 and B12. My body's natural detoxification ability is fast. This is the body's ability to detoxify itself of the free radicals which can be cell-harming, and are released when we eat smoked foods or chargrilled steak, for example. We have a natural ability to do that, but a diet full of anti- oxidants is also very helpful for detoxification.

Vitamin D3

My vitamin D3 levels came back as 'adequate', which was a little surprising given I spend a lot of time outdoors, and had a week in South Africa in January. That said, the test was taken in April when the UK is just coming out of winter, and if you're UK-based for most of the winter months, you'll be getting very little sun.

Adrenal stress levels

My adrenal stress levels were low, from waking to going to bed. I've explained that they should peak at time of waking, and then slowly decline until you go to bed. My levels were slightly lower than ideal upon waking, and then dropped quite rapidly before maintaining a low level until bedtime. This explained my waking patterns, as my cortisol levels were peaking too early in the day, and is also why I was waking up around 4.45am-5.15am and feeling so alert.

Basal body temperature

A healthy body temperature is 37° Celsius, or 98.6° Fahrenheit. The basal body temperature is a measure of your body's temperature when you wake. Mine was slightly lower than that, ranging from 35.9° to 36.4° Celsius. We had a suspicion that perhaps my thyroid was slightly underperforming, and agreed a short-term supplementation strategy followed by retesting to determine what was going on.

My therapeutic plan

The plan that was put together for me by my genetic nutritional expert was based around three objectives, which were to:

Recover my vitality and energy

Retrain the body's hormones via a specialised pattern of slow-releasing carbohydrates to support natural circadian rhythms and blood sugar balance

Replenish the nutrient stores depleted by stress through the abundant consumption of high-quality, nutrient-rich whole foods to support recovery and resilience

The main structure of the plan was to completely eliminate refined carbohydrates (of which sugar is one), all dairy products and all grains for 30 days. The diet isn't that dissimilar to the Paleo Diet if you are familiar with that. On the face of it, that seemed like quite a challenge, and indeed it was quite a while before I was able to get my head round it. Once I'd sat down and gone through it, working out what I could have and how that translated into a weekly food plan, it wasn't too difficult.

I was also given several supplements to support the new plan. These included iron tablets (for my low ferritin score), adrenal support tablets to help the adrenal glands recover, vitamin D3 (2500 IUs per day), and Pukka Clean Greens in tablet form.

My meals were structured around 30-40g of high-quality protein, 30-40g of healthy fats, and a very small amount of carbohydrate-rich foods such as a sweet potato (the amount varied according to which meal it was). I also had three portions of non-starchy vegetables such as greens. Snacks could include anything that was rich in healthy fats such as nuts, the occasional piece of fruit, and vegetables such as carrot sticks.

The 30-day elimination diet

The first week was, predictably, the hardest to get through, but in hindsight I could have made things easier for myself. I hadn't planned each meal for each day as thoroughly as I should have done. The planning itself is not a big deal, it's just about working out how to structure each meal, making sure the ingredients are in the house (and defrosted!), and that you have enough time to prepare and make the meal. My challenge was soon apparent; whilst I am highly motivated towards healthy eating, taking care of myself and being fit, my interests don't lie in the preparation and consideration of food. I love healthy, nutritious food, but I'm more interested in running a business and working face-to-face with clients than spending time in the kitchen preparing food. I'm still working on this adjustment to mindset, but if you're serious (as I am) about making these changes, then that's what has to be done.

The really startling thing was just how entrenched refined carbohydrates are in our society. There is almost nowhere on the high street that offers coffee, snacks and food, where the menu isn't almost entirely comprised of cakes, pastries, pasta, breads or potatoes. I can't pop out for a snack without really thinking about where I'll go. The downside of this is that if you haven't brought something with you like a Tupperware container full of nuts or fruit, then you'll go hungry or end up going 'off-piste' and eating refined carbs. That's something I realised quite quickly on this diet! The other thing I learned was also a surprise to me; that I actually rely on carbs for meals and snacks a lot more than I thought. It's only when you do something like a 30-day elimination diet that you recognise your patterns of eating. In that sense, it was a real eye-opener.

The second week was also hard, but I was better prepared and better organised. At home we drew up a meal plan on the Sunday before, and made sure we had all the food we needed in. It was also hard adjusting to the lack of carbs in my diet, and I felt really under-energised and quite weak in the gym. I spoke to the genetic nutritionist about whether I should increase my portions of non-starchy carbs by a little, but we both felt it was too early to judge as my body was still adapting to burning fat not carbs.

By the end of week two, I started to feel a bit more energised, and I noticed that my sleep was much better. I no longer woke early, and was able to sleep a bit later into the morning if I got the chance. I also used the ŌURA app to monitor my sleep, and it showed me that I was sleeping for longer, although still not regularly getting the eight hours sleep that I'd targeted.

It was during week three when I really started to feel better, and I would say totally adjusted to burning fat rather than carbohydrates. I still craved carbs, and had the odd sugar craving after a meal, but it was much better than it had been. I still had a challenge around getting enough healthy fats into breakfast, but found a solution by adding seeds and nuts into my morning green smoothie. As an experiment, I also started tracking my calories and food using an app, as I suspected there might be days when I burned more calories than I consumed. The calorie counting in the app isn't an exact science, but it confirmed what I thought: most days I consumed enough calories to match my expenditure, but on days where I trained harder than usual, there was a calorie deficit. Having access to this data meant I could revise my food plan for the day and get extra calories in on training days, which is essential for recovery and energy management.

By the end of week four, I felt much more comfortable with the new way of eating. I had fat-adapted for training, and I started to feel a bit lighter on my feet for running. I was waking up feeling clear-headed and feeling energised throughout the day. There were Pavlovian moments when I thought about (or had to look at other people eating) cakes or desserts, but the temptation to succumb to the desires just didn't hold much power over me. I was still taking the supplements, but phased these out over the following couple of weeks.

The reality of this is, that what can seem very complicated on paper is actually quite simple. The diet that I followed (read on to see if I've kept it up), is essentially just very healthy eating, with minimal sugar and other refined carbs, backed up by good quality supplements, lots of vegetables and plenty of protein and healthy fats. You can have the odd treat, but in moderation, and not in such a way that the body becomes disrupted by a dependency on refined carbs and sugar. I found it fairly easy to eliminate the sugar, dairy, grains and other refined carbs because I was very focused on finding out how I would feel without it. I wanted to know if I could feel better than this, and go back to my old boast of never getting sick instead of being bedridden by the 'mystery sickness' every two months.

Other thoughts and observations

There were three things that I found really fascinating during this exercise:

The first thing was discovering what it is like to be a client, and go through the kind of programme that we deliver. I can appreciate the challenges and obstacles that you have to go through, and how daunting it can seem at the start. I feel better equipped to have conversations with clients about what personalising their diet entails, and I can speak from personal experience and genuinely empathise with clients when they report how they're getting on.

The second observation was this: the power of cognitive dissonance and how easily fooled we are by ourselves. Cognitive dissonance is defined as 'the mental stress or discomfort experienced by an individual who holds two or more contradictory beliefs, ideas, or values at the same time'. Anyone who smokes, for example, is essentially practising cognitive dissonance because they know that smoking can seriously affect your health and can be fatal, but they enjoy it and carry on nonetheless. As a fitness professional, I know about the harmful effects of sugar, but still consciously consumed far too much. I was able to ignore it when it suited me, and let myself off by telling myself I was very lean and not getting fat, and I had no fillings so my teeth were unaffected. Cognitive dissonance. We all use it, but at some point we have to confront it and take action.

The third observation was just how much data we have at our disposal now, and how powerful it is. We are now living in an age where we have access to so much personal data, that technology can help us understand how we're performing and how we can improve on that performance. Whilst a lot of this – personalised nutrition, DNA testing, other tests, wearable tech – all comes with a price, it's there if we want to prioritise our health. You're reading this book, so you clearly care about your health and fitness. I urge you to go one step further and explore how you can personalise your lifestyle. Spend time (and if needed, money) now to get time back later.

How did personalising my diet help with my issues?

Let's go back to those initial issues.

Sugar cravings and overconsumption

Understanding the effects that sugar was having on my adrenals, appetite regulation and energy levels was highly motivating. Following a blood-sugar balancing diet that was low in GI and contained whole foods, including a lot of vegetables, protein, healthy fats and water helped to manage the cravings and eventually, the desire to have something sweet after a main meal disappeared. It did take several weeks though, and I had to work hard at not succumbing. The feeling of not being pulled around by an addiction or craving is a good one though, and I feel much happier knowing that I am pretty much sugar-free and am no longer using sugar as a reward.

Reflux and belching

It only took less than a week to notice that my reflux and belching had stopped almost completely. I now know that lactose was the main cause (along with carbohydrates) of both symptoms. I tried some innocently-named courgette fritters in a local restaurant and paid the price with both reflux and belching throughout the night as it turned out they were full of goat's cheese. That was a lesson learned! As a result, I've found the decision to give up lactose an easy one to make. I haven't gone back to large amounts of starchy carbs so I can't say for sure that they would cause either of the symptoms to recur, but I suspect they would. My DNA report states quite clearly that I am highly sensitive to carbs, and that matches my experience of consuming them.

Sleep

My sleep has definitely improved since changing my diet, and I monitor this based on how I feel when I wake up, and what the ŌURAring tells me. I do find it accurate, and it's interesting to match up how I feel with the pattern of sleep recorded by the app. Sometimes I feel rested, but the app shows I've been restless for several times a night. I've also made some adjustments to my nighttime routine to ensure a better night's sleep. For example, I drink a lot of herbal teas (not fruit teas as they contain sugar), and can almost chain-drink them in the evening. I find if I stop by around 9pm, I don't need to get up in the night to go to the toilet, which guarantees a better night's sleep. I have also banished my smartphone from the bedroom and gone back to using a good old-fashioned alarm clock. This keeps the device (and the potentially damaging electromagnetic fields) well clear of my head and it's impossible to reach out for it in the night if I can't sleep. I find I get a more restful and deep sleep if I read a book for 15-20 minutes before bed, so I try and make that my routine every night now.

The 'mystery sickness'

Perhaps not such a mystery after all! I think the cause was a combination of lactose overload, stress and overwork. Each of the sicknesses came at a time when there was a lot going on, but I don't think this would have been an issue had I been eating a diet that supported me well. What I was doing was fundamentally going against my genes – consuming high levels of refined carbs, saturated fat and lactose – so my body had a lot to cope with digesting these foods and trying to draw out some nutrition. I also think in hindsight that I was overtraining. My DNA report says I have a medium recovery profile, but often I would be repeating exercise sessions within 8-10 hours of the last one, therefore not allowing the body sufficient time to recover (or supporting it with the right diet). I used the DNA report to build in more rest in between sessions and dropped a couple of sessions from my weekly schedule. My strategy was to get more from doing less, and I feel that has worked well for me. I'm looking forward to my gym sessions, I have more energy and enthusiasm and because I'm more relaxed I'm getting better results. But it's not just about that; exercise is supposed to be enjoyable, not stressful. When it becomes stressful, you're either doing the wrong thing, or you're doing the right thing but overtraining. Symptoms of overtraining include loss of appetite, mood swings, tiredness that doesn't get better with a good night's sleep, anhedonia (a loss of pleasure where once you enjoyed something), irritability, broken sleep. I definitely had moments where these feelings were more than a passing phase, and that's almost certainly because I was overtraining, eating the wrong kind of diet, and trying to do too much.

> **Case Study - the expert's view**
>
> Note this section is quite technical, so if you are less interested in the details then please turn to chapter 9.

Symptoms

Dysregulated sleep pattern (waking at 4:15-5:30am with energy, lethargic when wakes again at 7am, occasional disturbed sleep earlier in night); instances every two months of mystery sickness lasting three days with dry retching, lethargy, achy legs and limbs, and mild aversion to light, requiring complete bed rest for recovery; frequent, persistent cough for years, especially upon waking, and with a lowered lung capacity; frequent belching, especially after meals and if carbohydrate-heavy; frequent acid reflux that is worse at night; regular bloating in lower abdomen; bowel movement one to two times per day of Bristol Stool Type 3-4; night sweats; bloating monthly prior to menstrual cycle; frequent, intense sugar cravings mid-day and after evening meal; medium dry skin; yellow coating on tongue; stress levels average at around five out of 10.

Medications/Medical History

Has just completed several months of daily lansoprazole therapy; preventative regular use of brown steroid inhaler; has been diagnosed with asthma but believes this could be an inaccurate diagnosis.

Test Results

DNAFit Key Polymorphisms: high carbohydrate sensitivity; medium fat sensitivity; high saturated fat sensitivity; GSTM1 deletion; homozygous slow enzymatic activity SOD2, CAT, CYP1A2; heterozygous GPX1, VDR, IL6; lactose intolerant.

DNAFit Functional Analysis: reduce overall carbohydrate intake; minimise/eliminate grains; eliminate refined carbohydrates; moderate unsaturated fat intake; limit saturated fat intake; eliminate dairy (other than small amounts of ghee, which potentially may not cause reaction); phase II liver detoxification down-regulation; significantly increased sensitivity to oxidative stress; moderately increased predisposition to inflammation; raised nutrient requirements for vitamin D, omega-3, antioxidants, selenium, indole-3-carbinoles (cruciferous vegetables).

Vitamin D: 89.9 nmol/L

Adrenal Stress Profile:moderately reduced waking cortisol; somewhat reduced mid-morning and afternoon cortisol; raised evening cortisol; low morning DHEA; borderline DHEA: cortisol ratio.

Adrenal Profile Functional Analysis is progressing from the initial 'stressed' phase of adrenal gland hyper-production to following 'wired and tired' stage.

Key systems under stress

Gastrointestinal Tract:

bloating; burping; yellow tongue coating; lactose intolerance; acid reflux; possible dysbiosis; reduced bowel elimination.

Nervous System:

dysregulated sleep pattern; moderate stress levels.

Endocrine System:

dysregulated adrenal gland function; night sweats; high sugar cravings.

Respiratory:

persistent cough; lowered lung capacity.

Assessment of key underlying drivers and symptom development

The body and digestive system is being put under pressure through a combination of high sugar intake, dairy consumption, stress, reduced liver detoxification, imbalanced omega-3 and dietary fat intake, and inadequate dietary antioxidant intake. Hormones produced by stress further increase the stress load on already overburdened systems. There is also a gut microbiome imbalance, sub-optimal digestive function, and lactose intolerance. All have been further compounded by sustained moderate stress levels, the effect of which can also be seen in the poor regulation of stress hormones.

This has led to a distinct combination of symptoms. First, the recurring mystery sickness every two months, the result of the body's natural detoxification and oxidative stress management systems reaching a tipping point, enforcing a period of rest and lowered metabolic function. Second, a persistent immune imbalance presenting in respiratory symptoms and lowered lung capacity.

Recovery plan and aims

1. Support adrenal function: adjust and rebalance carbohydrate consumption; eliminate refined carbohydrate and grains; adrenal glandular supplementation; optimise dietary nutrient intake for co-factor support.

2. Optimise digestive function: eliminate dairy, adjust and rebalance carbohydrate consumption; eliminate refined carbohydrate and grains.

3. Lower oxidative stress and rebalance immune system: eliminate dairy, adjust and rebalance carbohydrate consumption; eliminate refined carbohydrate and grains; increase dietary antioxidant intake; increase omega-3 intake; probiotic supplementation; limit saturated fat consumption.

4. Support detoxification: increase frequency of bowel motility; daily cruciferous vegetables intake; increase dietary fibre.

Chapter 9:
Empowerment and Inspiration

Superhuman self-belief

Whilst I was writing this book, I witnessed two events which really inspired me, one in person and the other on television. I love witnessing people perform incredible feats of strength and daring; challenging themselves both physically and mentally and achieving things that most people couldn't dream of. I find it both exhilarating, and very motivational. I believe that when other people stretch themselves beyond their imaginations, it rubs off on others. There is nothing more exciting than pushing yourself beyond your expectations and seeing what you can achieve without limitations.

Eddie Izzard and Sport Relief

The first arrow of inspiration was a television programme. It was a Sport Relief programme about Eddie Izzard's attempt to run 27 marathons in 27 days. He chose 27 because that was the number of years that Nelson Mandela was incarcerated in South Africa, and the route he took was also a retracing of Mandela's childhood and upbringing.

I've run two marathons, and they were two years apart. For those of you who haven't run one, a marathon is a very long way. It's a cliché to say it's a journey, but it really is. You go through a whole gamut of emotions, from elation to euphoria, to misery and pain. Setting aside the matter of the combined 707.4 miles, the psychological and mental strength you need to possess to even consider such an undertaking is something that few of us can imagine. Knowing that day after day you'll be running 26.2 miles in temperatures of up to 40°, with no rest day, is a heavy psychological burden to carry. Running just a single marathon requires mental strength. Added to that, Izzard had attempted the same feat in 2012 but had to pull out after the third marathon because his muscles were breaking down, making his pee a dark brown colour. He was clearly anxious about getting past marathon number three and ridding himself of any perceived jinx.

He did have setbacks and niggles, including a few trips to the same hospital he'd ended up in before, but exactly 27 days after he'd started, Izzard crossed the final finish line and staggered to the Nelson Mandela statue in Pretoria. It was a poignant end to the journey, and Izzard looked humbled and happy to be collapsed at the feet of his idol, a man who has inspired so many of us and continues to do so. During filming, Izzard talked briefly about other adversities he'd had to overcome in his life, not least the taunting, bullying and animosity he'd faced having come out as a transgender man 31 years ago. I have tremendous respect for him and what he stands for; his strength, unerring focus, resilience and principles.

Circa at the Udderbelly on the Southbank

The Udderbelly is a crazy upside-down purple cow that resides on London's Southbank for the spring and summer months, next to the London Eye. A small group of circus performers – athletes who perform astonishing feats of strength, flexibility and daring – entertain for a little over an hour using chairs, a trapeze, bodyweight and hula hoops (lots of them). I love anything that shows off what the human body can do if trained and nurtured, and this show is a feast for like-minds. The most striking aspect of what they do is the level of trust between the five performers; they have each other's backs, and they know it, so when they jump, leap or climb on each other, they know they will be secure.

It's a great example of what happens when people work together. Almost every scene features at least two performers, working in synchronicity and fluidity. It's timed to perfection, but you still find yourself gasping as one makes their move, or sitting in silent suspense just in case a twitch or tremor by someone in the audience distracts them. If you want to see what the human body can do, when the mind is as sharply trained as theirs are, and courage is in abundance, then go and see this show.

The other interesting thing for me was their physiques. Each performer was as strong as an ox, capable of carrying a person on their shoulders, and sometimes more. What they could endure from a physical perspective was beyond belief. But with the exception of one performer, none of them were what you would call 'ripped'. Their bodies had been trained to be strong and enduring, not cut and chiseled into the types of bodies you see on advertisement billboards. These bodies have been trained for functional fitness not aesthetics, and that made them all the more extraordinary to me. No 'muscle man' or 'bikini body' about these bodies, just pure strength.

I've been lifted by both these events, and it's made me consider what I want to do next to challenge myself, whether it's in fitness or business, or something completely different. I think it's important to regularly challenge yourself; consider what you'll do to stretch yourself and push past your limitations. Be brave.

Making connections

I had the pleasure of meeting Dame Kelly Holmes for a few minutes, and I really warmed to her. Her story is inspirational, and she came across as a very humble, funny person. Underneath that though lies a will of steel; she said despite the difficulties of her upbringing, all she focused on was becoming the best athlete she could be, and for her it was being an Olympian. She also talked very openly about her depression, and how she overcame that, which was touching to hear and generous of her to be so open. What an incredible woman.

A sense of connection

Later that day, I was at a Dixie Chicks concert at the O2. Already feeling good about meeting the Dame, I thought the day couldn't get much better. I don't like crowds of people, and was slightly unsettled at the thought of going to the O2 as it's such a vast venue, but I had one of the best times of my life at a concert. The Chicks were brilliant, and despite the very diverse range of people there, I've never felt such a sense of connection anywhere. We sang our hearts out (I have a poor singing voice but it was too loud for anyone to notice), friends were hugging, small children were rocking out and everyone young and old was there to have a good time. It was a wonderful feeling to be a part of the wholeness made up of tens of thousands of very different people and I'm still buzzing from it. It really made me think of the power that occurs when a group of people get together with a common interest or purpose, and how important it is to connect with people. It also reminded me of something I'd forgotten; how music unites us all and has the power to lift our spirits.

The power of connecting

If you haven't felt that sense of connection for a while, try and create that feeling for yourself (and others). It might only be a small group of friends going out for an evening or for a walk in the countryside.

It might even be just one person. But if you feel that connection, you'll feel amazing. It's a basic human need. Brené Brown defines human connection as this:

"The energy that exists between people when they feel seen, heard, and valued; when they can give and receive without judgment; and when they derive sustenance and strength from the relationship."

Finding like-minded people makes us feel good; we like to see aspects of ourselves reflected back in others, it's reassuring and comforting. Connections can be made in other, more personal, ways too. You can form a deep connection with your body, through breathing techniques, yoga and exercise. It's important to connect with your goals, and your intent; why are you doing something, what's your purpose and how do you want to feel afterwards?

Connecting with your purpose

I think this is very important. There's our broader life purpose, or the purpose which drives our work. My purpose is to help clients prolong their healthspan through the promotion of personalised diet and exercise. This defines much of what I do and is my 'why'. I love doing that. Take some time out to consider what your purpose is, and then reverse engineer this to work out what your intent is each day. You'll find you're much more efficient in what you do if this is clear to you. Humans were designed to solve meaningful problems; we were made to move; we have evolved to respond to the challenges put in front of us, often of our own making. We need a clear purpose, a clear intent, and without it we lose that sense of connection.

Seven habits of consistently fit people

I've spent a lot of time with people of different fitness levels, with their own set of challenges and preoccupations. Some people identify the connection between exercise and the feeling of being fit, and form lasting habits that mean they can sustain their fitness; they naturally associate physical fitness with overall wellbeing. Others struggle to get into a rhythm and find themselves exercising and dieting in a rollercoaster cycle of up and down, which can be quite mentally exhausting. Having spent a few years running a health and fitness consultancy, as well as following a very consistent and disciplined exercise regime myself, I've observed the traits and behavioural patterns that consistently fit people display. It's important to mention that it's not about any individual thing, but more about how you can blend these traits to develop that consistency.

1. They don't rely on guesswork

    There is now a wide range of wearable technology that can tell you how you're performing in different types of exercise. There are also apps that enable you to track what you're eating, and ensure you're getting the right amount of nutrients within a balanced diet. A DNA test can tell you what your requirements are for key vitamins and minerals; your sensitivity to lactose, gluten, carbohydrates and saturated fat; and what the best type of exercise is for you based on your genes. The test will also tell you what your recovery, injury risk and VO2 Max trainability is. Training according to your genetic profile, and monitoring results, helps to maintain a consistent training programme with minimal risk of injury and setbacks.

2. **They know when to increase training loads and when to rest.**

   This is really important. You must listen to your body, and learn to read the signals it sends you and then have the discipline to respond to those signals and messages. Some of my most notable improvements to strength and fitness have come after a period of reduced training and increased rest. To some this might seem paradoxical, but many of us are now living, working and training under quite extreme stress. We're juggling many different facets of our lives, and sometimes we can become overwhelmed without realising it. The body keeps the score, and ignoring the warning signs can be counterproductive to your health and fitness.

3. **They have an active body and an active mind**

   I have yet to meet anyone who has a consistent diet and exercise programme who isn't a very active person, mentally and physically. They read, whether it's online or print, novels or newspapers. They question, and are naturally curious about things. They want to move, to explore, and to challenge themselves. They will instinctively take the stairs instead of the escalator. I encourage you to set yourselves an annual or biannual challenge; something that terrifies you. It's really healthy to take yourself out of your comfort zone every now and then and see what you're capable of. Get comfortable being uncomfortable as they say. Your self-esteem and self-confidence will soar.

4. **They are used to setting SMART goals**

   SMART goals are Simple, Measurable, Achievable, Realistic and Time-bound. I often see people fail because the goals they set themselves were too tough. Start small, then build on your progress. This applies to dieting and exercise. Any diet that cuts out a key food group or involves a dramatic calorie reduction for example, is doomed to failure. We advise our clients to identify three aspects of their diet to work on, and take the time required to interweave those changes into their lifestyle. Once that's achieved, look to another three things. I have many examples of where that strategy has been a roaring success. Set SMART goals and ask someone else who knows you well and is supportive of what you're doing to review them for you.

5. They see the bigger picture

A sustainable (and therefore successful) diet and exercise programme requires you to see the bigger picture. People who achieve consistent success in this area understand that good health can be put down to many different things. To give you an idea, some of these things include managing stress, getting into a good sleep routine, having rules around your smartphone and computer at night, maintaining healthy relationships, hydration, having good self-esteem, eating a balanced diet, knowing when to train and when to rest, walking regularly, remembering to laugh, doing a job you like (if not love) and that is authentic to you.

6. They know when to enlist help

Everyone has times when they need a boost, a bit of motivation, and maintaining the consistency sometimes means enlisting outside help. Hiring a fitness coach to retain focus wouldn't be unusual for this type of person, nor would recruiting the services of a nutritionist or a life coach. All these things cost money, and usually the really good people will be expensive, but what price is your health? I consider myself to be a very disciplined and motivated person; I co-run a very successful and rapidly-growing health and fitness consultancy; I've planned, written and published my first book in less than six months, and launched a new brand of fitness coaching to help executives recover from burnout. Despite this, I still have the same personal trainer I've had for nine years to keep me motivated and put me through my paces three times a week. Why? Because we all need help sometimes, and you simply don't push yourself as hard as someone else will.

7. **They know what works for them**

Are you a lone wolf or pack animal? People who manage to maintain a consistent diet and exercise regime understand what kind of exercise works well for them (and it isn't a chore). If you love classes, and get a buzz from working out with others and pitting yourself against them, don't set SMART goals which mean you're spending a lot of time on your own. If you prefer a long, solitary run, build your regime around that. If you're getting a buzz out of what you're doing, your brain will naturally propel you into repeating that activity. That said, never be afraid to try something new, but if you've given it a few tries and it's not working for you, then move on.

Find Your Purpose

I'm often asked why I left a well-paid job in the City to start working as a fitness entrepreneur. It's a good question. I had no clients, no equipment, no logo, no branding, just a Diploma in Personal Training (it takes six weeks to attain that qualification – frightening, isn't it?). I had gone from a guaranteed income which permitted a good lifestyle, with a team of people to do things for me, to a situation where if I didn't make it happen, it wasn't going to happen. I loved it.

Why? Because I knew I could create something special given time. I knew that I had something that was crucial for success, a thing that would enable me to attract clients, a team, partners and opportunities; a sense of purpose.

My purpose

My purpose in life and in business is this: I want to empower people to prolong their healthspan by reigniting lives, strengthening bodies and empowering minds. This drives both Bodyshot Performance® and The RISE Method®. What we do far transcends fitness coaching. Our role is to be a change agent, building a relationship with our clients that extends into every day, not just the days we're together. We need to be unafraid to challenge clients when they need challenging, and to avoid over-praising, which can hinder progress.

So if it's not about fitness coaching, what's it really about?

It's about asking the right questions, timing, emotional intelligence, pacing, and above all, listening.

It's about breaking negative habits and freeing our clients to live happier lives.

It's about helping people reconnect with their bodies.

It's about helping people open their minds to the power of human movement

It's about empowering clients to take responsibility for their health and to realise their dreams.

It's about making the connections between movement, health and fulfilling our potential.

So if you think it's all about fitness coaching, then you've missed the point. It's about so much more than nutrition, exercise and motivation. Our clients go on to achieve great things once they've made the connection between movement, health and potential. If you aren't there yet, start today. Go out for a walk or a short jog. Stir up the basic human need for movement and feel the blood rushing through your body.

Find your purpose.

My Predictions For Future Fitness Trends

I strongly believe that the times we live in now are very exciting for the health and fitness industry, and therefore for our clients as well. Most of the trends I've outlined in this post have a common theme: **personalisation**, which is what this book has been all about. If you follow these trends, you too could see greater results for potentially the same amount of effort. Here are my predictions for the next 12 to 18 months:

Wearable technology

Gadgets such as the Apple Watch, Garmin, Jawbone, Fitbit and Nike Bands have been out for a while now, and there are even virtual reality headsets that you can use whilst exercising. We're seeing more and more clients wearing these gadgets, and there's definitely more interest in tracking health-related data amongst the people I come into contact with. Devices such as the ŌURAring are now overtaking the more outdated devices by adding in intelligent analysis. I predict that we will see even more people buying devices that can help them understand how much they're moving, and what effect it's having on their fitness.

Tapping into your DNA

Genetic tests can now identify the ideal diet type and best type of exercise for each individual. This science is revolutionising the fitness world, and removes the educated guesswork that happens otherwise. The one-size-fits-all approach is now outdated. Want to know what your carbohydrate and saturated fat sensitivity is, or whether you have a requirement for cruciferous vegetables and anti-oxidants? Or whether you're better suited to power or endurance, and what your injury risk and recovery times are? Your DNA can now provide the answers.

Leaving the gym for outdoor training

I predict that more people will want to train outside, as opposed to working out in a sweaty gym. Boot Camps have seen a huge uptake in recent years, and I believe this is largely because they are (usually) held outdoors, and give people a chance to run around in the fresh air. Most of us work indoors, and in winter months, you can leave the house in darkness, and return in darkness, therefore seeing very little natural light or fresh air. Working out outdoors, once you've got over the cold, can be very liberating and make you feel less confined.

Using a fitness coach

As time becomes ever more precious, and our lives seem to get busier, a lot of people are now looking to an expert to help them maximise their time spent exercising. I predict that fitness coaching will become even more popular in 2016, as people look to get the best results they can in the time they spend exercising. Carl Benedikt-Frey (Co-Director of the Oxford Martin Programme on Technology and Employment at the University of Oxford) stated "the fastest-growing occupations in the past five years are all related to services. The two biggest are Zumba instructor and personal trainer."

Using exercise as a form of therapy

We have long known the benefits of exercise on mental health, but I think 2016 will see a lot more people taking up exercise to help them with problems affecting mental health such as stress, anxiety and depression. I am a big advocate of using exercise to help with mental health, and issues such as professional burnout and stress in the workplace are becoming more widely discussed and appreciated. Several large firms now have mental health champions, and a number of firms of all sizes have schemes designed to help people manage stress at work, and all these schemes encourage exercise in one form or another.

Older adults

Awareness of the need to exercise and stay mobile is increasing now in older adults, with an increasing number of older people attending specialist classes and using the parks to stay fit. I've seen an increase in the number of older adults who have come to us for fitness coaching; often they are looking for help reducing their cholesterol or blood pressure, but they also want to strengthen their muscles, ligaments and tendons to reduce the risk of falling. Older women are also aware of the need to exercise to strengthen their bones and reduce the risk of osteoporosis.

Yoga

I predict that yoga will become even more popular in the next 12 months. New styles of yoga are cropping up, such as BoxingYoga™, which blends elements of a fighter's training with classic vinyasa flow yoga moves. Traditional forms of yoga still remain very popular, and more people are developing an appreciation for what yoga brings to the body and mind. I believe that yoga is a great complement to any other form of exercise, where usually the focus is on shortening the muscles rather than lengthening and stretching. Yoga can help mitigate the risk of injury, as well as keeping you supple and relaxed.

Ten Maxims for a Healthy and Happy Life

1. The world needs diversity. Be different, be brave, be adventurous

2. Fear drives a lot of negative behaviours. Find a way to be unafraid

3. Nurture your talents, they will set you apart from others

4. Most people settle for being average. Make your life surprising and remarkable

5. Life will be full of challenges sometimes; it's how you deal with them that matters

6. Be free to love who you want, as long as they're worthy of you

7. The world needs strong, independent, driven women; embrace this maxim

8. Be brave, truthful and never shy away from doing the right thing

9. Don't be too proud to ask for help if you need it, It's not weakness

10. Make the most of every second because there's so much life to be lived

Glossary

Allelle – each of two or more alternative forms of a gene that arise by mutation and are found at the same place on a chromosome. Also called *allelomorph*

Adrenal hormone – *endocrine glands* that produce a variety of hormones including *adrenaline* and the steroids *aldosterone* and *cortisol*.[1] They are found above the *kidneys*

Anti-oxidants – man-made or natural substances that may prevent or delay some types of cell damage. Antioxidants are found in many foods, including fruits and vegetables. They are also available as dietary supplements

Catecholamines – any of a class of aromatic amines which includes a number of neurotransmitters such as adrenaline and dopamine

Cirdadian rhythms – a daily cycle of biological activity based on a 24-hour period and influenced by regular variations in the environment, such as the alternation of night and day

Cortisol – a steroid hormone, in the glucocorticoid class of hormones. It is released in response to stress and low blood-glucose concentration

Cruciferous vegetables – *vegetables* of the family *Brassicaceae* (also called Cruciferae). These vegetables are widely cultivated, with many genera, species, and cultivars being raised for food production such as *cauliflower, cabbage, garden cress, bok choy, broccoli, brussels sprouts* and similar green-leaf vegetables

Detoxification – the metabolic process by which toxins are changed into less toxic or more readily excretable substances

Dopamine – a neurotransmitter. It is a chemical messenger that helps in the transmission of signals in the brain and other vital areas

Endorphins – the body's natural opiates, designed to relieve stress and enhance pleasure

Epigenetics – the study, in the field of genetics, of cellular and physiological phenotypic trait variations that are caused by external or environmental factors that switch genes on and off and affect how cells read genes

Epinephrine – another term for *adrenaline*

Fast-twitch – (of a muscle fibre) contracting rapidly, thus providing strength rather than endurance

Genotype – the genetic constitution of an individual organism. Often contrasted with *phenotype*

Gluten – is a mixture of *proteins* found in *wheat* and related grains, including *barley, rye,*[1] *oat,*[2] and all their species and hybrids

Gluteus Medius – one of the three *gluteal muscles,* is a broad, thick, radiating muscle, situated on the outer surface of the *pelvis*

HIIT – an acronym for high intensity interval training

Hippocampus – region of the brain that is associated primarily with *memory*

Hypertrophy – the increase in the volume of an organ or tissue due to the enlargement of its component cells. It is distinguished from hyperplasia, in which the cells remain approximately the same size but increase in number

Hyponatremia – also called water intoxication, is generally the result of drinking excessive amounts of plain water which causes a low concentration of *sodium* in the blood

Ischial tuberosity – known informally as the sitz bone, or as a pair the sitting bones

ITB (iliotibial band) – a thick band of *fascia* on the lateral aspect of the knee, extending from the outside of the *pelvis*, over the *hip* and knee, and inserting just below the knee

Lactose – *a disaccharide sugar* derived from *galactose* and *glucose* that is found in *milk*

Microbiome – the microorganisms in a particular environment (including the body or a part of the body

Mitochondria – a double *membrane*-bound *organelle* found in all *eukaryotic* organisms

Morphogenetic – the biological process that causes an organism to develop its shape. It is one of three fundamental aspects of developmental biology along with the control of cell growth and cellular differentiation, unified in evolutionary developmental biology

Neurogenesis – the process by which neurons are generated from neural stem cells and progenitor cells. It plays a central role in neural development

Neurotransmitters – also known as chemical messengers, are *endogenous chemicals* that enable *neurotransmission*. They transmit signals across a *chemical synapse*, such as a *neuromuscular junction*, from one *neuron* (nerve cell) to another "target" neuron, *muscle cell*, or *gland cell*

Norepinephrine – also called noradrenaline or noradrenalin, is an organic chemical in the catecholamine family that functions in the human brain and body as a hormone and neurotransmitter

Nucleus – the central and most important part of an object, movement, or group, forming the basis for its activity and growth

Obesogenic – tending to cause obesity

Omega-3 – also called ω-3 fatty acids or n-3 fatty acids — are polyunsaturated fatty acids with a double bond at the third carbon atom from the end of the carbon chain

ŌURAring – ring-sized wearable technology that collects activity and inactivity data and cross-correlates it against sleep data to provide personalised insights to improve performance

Oxidative stress – reflects an imbalance between the systemic manifestation of *reactive oxygen species* and a biological system's ability to readily *detoxify* the reactive intermediates or to repair the resulting damage

Phenotype – the set of observable characteristics of an individual resulting from the interaction of its genotype with the environment

Polymorphisms – the condition of occurring in several different forms

Proteins – *large biomolecules*, or *macromolecules*, consisting of one or more long chains of *amino acid residues*. Proteins perform a vast array of functions within *organisms*, including *catalysing metabolic reactions*, *DNA replication*, *responding to stimuli*, and *transporting molecules* from one location to another

Receptors – an organ or cell able to respond to light, heat, or other external stimulus and transmit a signal to a sensory nerve

Serotonin – a chemical found in the human body. It carries signals along and between nerves (a neurotransmitter)

Single Nucleotide Polymorphism (SMP) – a variation in a single nucleotide that occurs at a specific position in the genome, where each variation is present to some appreciable degree within a population

[1]**Slow-twitch** – (of a muscle fibre) contracting slowly, providing endurance rather than strength

Tabata – a 4-minute exercise sequence that is comprised of 8 repetitions of 20 seconds of intense exercise followed by 10 seconds of rest

Vasodilation – the constriction of blood vessels, which increases blood pressure

Vasodilation – Vasodilation refers to the widening of blood vessels. It results from relaxation of smooth muscle cells within the vessel walls, in particular in the large veins, large arteries, and smaller arterioles

Appendix A:
The Genes

Angiotensin I-converting enzyme (ACE)

ACE is a small enzyme that plays an important role in blood pressure regulation and electrolyte balance. Its activity leads to blood vessel constriction and increased blood pressure. The variation tested is the Insertion (I) / Deletion (D) variation in which a piece of DNA is either present or deleted from the gene. The (I) allele (an allele is one of a number of alternative forms of the same gene) is associated with lower ACE activity. This is the most researched gene in relation to sporting performance.

Adrenoceptor Beta 2 (Arg16Gly)

ADRB2 Beta (2)-adrenergic receptors are expressed throughout the body and serve as receptors for the natural stimulant hormones called catecholamines, or more specifically, epinephrine (adrenaline) and norepinephrine. The polymorphisms tested result in aminoacid changes, which affect the activity of the receptor and alter the response to these hormones. Beta- adrenergic receptors are found in fat cells, liver and skeletal muscle where they are involved in fat mobilization, blood glucose levels and in vasodilation.

Adrenoceptor Beta 2 (Gln27Glu)

ADRB2 Beta (2)-adrenergic receptors are expressed throughout the body and serve as receptors for the natural stimulant hormones called catecholamines epinephrine (adrenaline) and norepinephrine.

The polymorphisms tested result in amino acid changes, which affect the activity of the receptor and alter the response to these hormones. Beta-adrenergic receptors are found in fat cells, liver and skeletal muscle where they are involved in fat mobilization, blood glucose levels and in vasodilation.

Apolipoprotein A-II (APOA2)

Apolipoprotein A-II is a component of HDL particles where it is the second most abundant protein – its exact function though is not yet known but it is associated with obesity risk and type of food intake. The SNP tested is in the promoter of the gene so may affect levels of the protein. Studies repeated in several ethnic groups showed that the genetic variation can affect BMI but only when saturated fat in the diet is high.

Fatty Acid Binding Protein 2 (FABP2)

This protein is found only in cells of the small intestine, the main site for fat absorption and FABP2 is involved in the uptake and transport of both saturated and unsaturated fatty acids. The polymorphism tested for causes an amino acid change from Alanine to Threonine at position 54 in the protein sequence, and this version has a two-fold higher affinity for long-chain fatty acids. The Thr54 version is associated with increased fat oxidation and studies have shown that Thr54 may increase fat uptake in the small intestine – for example, it has been shown that after a fatty meal the levels of triglycerides in the blood are higher in Thr/Thr individuals. The Thr allele has also been linked to higher levels of total cholesterol and LDL cholesterol and lower levels of HDL (so called "good" cholesterol).

Fat Mass and Obesity Associated (FTO)FTO is a protein that is associated with fat mass and obesity in both adults and children. Its function has not been completely determined yet. It is an alpha-ketoglutarate- dependent deoxygenase enzyme that repairs alkylated DNA and RNA by oxidative demethylation (DNA, or deoxyribonucleic acid, is like a blueprint of biological guidelines that a living organism must follow to exist and remain functional. RNA, or ribonucleic acid, helps carry out this blueprint's guidelines). Activity appears to be affected by eating and fasting. The enzyme is particularly active in areas of the brain that are associated with eating behaviour.

Peroxisome Proliferator-Activated Receptor Gamma (PPARG)

This long-named protein is a receptor found in the cell nucleus – PPARG is important in the formation and development of adipocytes (fat cells). As a nuclear receptor when certain molecules bind to it (e.g. prostaglandins) it can itself bind directly to DNA and influence the expression of specific genes. In this way it regulates fatty acid storage and glucose metabolism. The SNP tested changes the amino acid at position 12 in the protein from Proline to Alanine, and the Ala version has a reduced affinity for target genes, this means it binds to them less strongly and has a reduced effect on their expression. The Ala form seems to have a protective effect against higher BMI and also reduced insulin sensitivity, but only under certain conditions.

Adrenoceptor Beta 3 (ADRB3)

Beta (3)-adrenergic receptors are located mainly in adipose tissue and they play a key role in energy metabolism, being involved in the regulation of lipolysis (fat breakdown) and thermogenesis (process of heat generation using fat for energy). The polymorphism that is tested results in an amino acid change from tryptophan (Trp) to Arginine (Arg) and the Arg version is associated with lower fat breakdown activity. (A polymorphism is a term used to describe multiple forms of a single gene that exists). Some studies have shown that the Arg allele is associated with a high BMI and that Arg allele carriers have more difficulty losing weight under standard weight loss diet and exercise protocols. The Arg allele has also been shown in studies to be linked to more rapid weight gain following dieting.

Transcription Factor 7-Like 2 (TCF7L2)

TCF7L2 is a transcription factor (a protein which binds to DNA and affects the expression of genes and the amount of various proteins produced) – it affects a variety of genes. It has not been fully characterised but the protein has been implicated in blood glucose homeostasis and the SNP tested affects insulin sensitivity. The polymorphism has also been shown to affect weight loss according to diet type with the TT homozygotes responding poorly to high fat/low carb diets. The T allele may also make weight loss harder with standard diet and exercise protocols and it is associated with increased weight gain after dieting. While the T allele, and in particular the TT genotype is linked to negative insulin/glucose balance the good news is that these effects can be neutralised by the correct diet, reducing weight if overweight and regular exercise.

Peroxisome Proliferator-Activated Receptor Alpha (PPARA)

Regulates genes responsible for skeletal and heart muscle fatty acid oxidation and is a main regulator of energy metabolism.

Vitamin D Receptor (VDR)

Associated with Vitamin D3 levels in the blood. Vitamin D3 is involved in maintaining appropriate calcium and phosphorous levels in the blood and providing immune support.

Alpha Actinin 3 (ACTN3)

Associated with a major structural component of the fast-twitch fibres of skeletal muscles. Only present in fast-twitch muscle fibres.

Peroxisome Proliferator-Activated Receptor Gamma Coactivator-1 (PPARGC1A)

Associated with the regulation of energy homeostasis, including production of mitochondria (an organelle found in large numbers in most cells, in which the biochemical processes of respiration and energy production occur). Also associated with fat and carbohydrate burning and conversion of muscle fibres to slow twitch type.

C-Reactive Protein (CRP)

Associated with an acute phase protein which rises in response to inflammation in the body. High CRP is associated with low VO2MAX (VO2 Max is the measure of how efficiently the body can take in oxygen). Diet and physical activity can reduce CRP levels (although intense exercise can cause short term local increases in CRP). It is stimulated by IL-6 and is often used as a marker for inflammation in blood tests.

Angiotensinogen (AGT)

Associated with vasoconstriction and blood pressure control.

Collagen 1 Alpha 1 (COL1A1)

Associated with vasodilation, blood pressure control, efficiency of muscular contraction and cell hydration.

Interleukin-6 - a pro- inflammatory cytokine (IL-6)

Stimulates the immune response to training and is involved in the inflammatory repair process.

Collagen 5 Alpha 1 (COL5A1)

Associated with Alpha-1 chain of type V collagen.

Growth Differentiation Factor 5 (GDF5)

Associated with a bone morphogenetic protein involved in joint formation, and with the Central Nervous System expression and the healing of skeletal, joint and soft tissues.

Thyrotrophin Releasing Hormone Receptor (TRHR)

Associated with regulation of the metabolic rate, mobilisation of fuels during exercise and also growth of lean body tissue.

Glutathione S-transferase M1 and T1 (GSTM1, GSTT1)

Associated with the removal of toxins, metabolic by-products, and free radicals created during the detoxification process.

Acknowledgments

Big thanks go to my eagle-eyed proofreaders who read the manuscript for me and picked up on lots of things that I'd missed: thanks to my Mum, Carolyn Walsham, old pal Sam Heckford and our right-hand woman Emma Bibby for your help with this book.

I'd also like to thank my publishers, Lucy and Joe at Rethink Press, for their hard work in getting this to print quickly and to such a high standard. Thank you to Andrew and Daniel Priestley and the KPI community who are always such as inspiration, and who encouraged me to write my first book and therefore become addicted to the writing process.

Lastly, a big thank you to my partner Antonia, who makes sure everything gets done at home whilst I shut myself off to write, and to our ageing cats Monty and Maddie for their calming presence.

The Author

Leanne Spencer is a fitness entrepreneur, author of the bestselling book *Rise and Shine: Recover from burnout and get back to your best*, and co-founder of Bodyshot Performance Limited. Bodyshot is a fast-growing disruptor in the fitness world; we combine your unique DNA, highly sophisticated wearable technology and bespoke coaching to transform the lives of our clients.

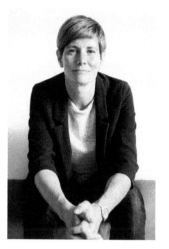

Leanne began her career in the City working for various companies as an Account Director. In 2012, after suffering from burnout, she resigned from her job and set about completely changing her career, lifestyle and mindset. After a period of rest and recovery, Leanne and her business partner created the health and fitness consultancy that is now called Bodyshot Performance Limited. Bodyshot have worked with hundreds of clients to help them understand how to adapt their lifestyle to get the best out of themselves.

Remove the Guesswork is Leanne's second book, but won't be her last as she finds the writing process quite addictive. Leanne also regularly blogs for a leading brand accelerator as well as on her own website (www.bodyshotperformance.com), and is a sharp and engaging speaker on topics relating to health, fitness, entrepreneurship, lifestyle, purpose, empowerment and inspiration, diet, exercise, burnout and stress, anxiety and depression. She also contributes articles to business and entrepreneurial magazines as well as fitness magazines. You can connect with Leanne via Twitter using the handle @BodyshotPT or Facebook by typing in Bodyshot Performance Limited, or send an email with any questions you might have to leanne@bodyshotperformance.com.

Leanne lives in South London with her partner and two cats, but escapes to the countryside and to sunnier climes whenever possible.

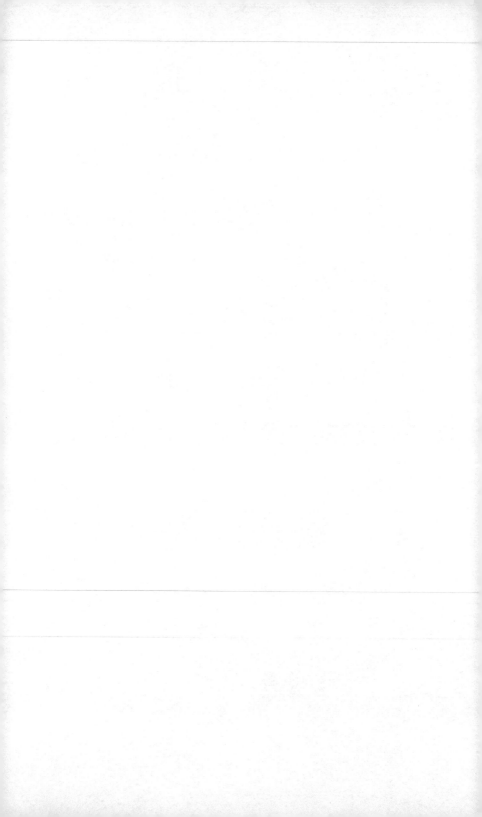